Thriving in
Unpredictable Times

Thriving in Unpredictable Times

A reader on 'agility' in health care

edited by

Sarah W. Fraser, Maxine Conner, David Yarrow

First published in 2003
by Kingsham Press

Oldbury Complex
Marsh Lane
Easthampnett
Chichester, West Sussex
PO18 OJW
United Kingdom

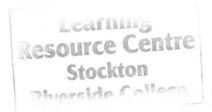

Typeset in AGaramond

Printed and bound by
Antony Rowe Ltd
Chippenham
Wiltshire
United Kingdom

ISBN: 1-904235-10-7

British Library Cataloging in Publication Data
A catalogue record of this book is available from the British Library

Fraser, Sarah; Conner, Maxine; Yarrow, David.

Contents

About the authors

Ruth Adam is project manager for Brent Older Peoples Project. Prior to the project Ruth was involved in developing the Collaborative Care Team based at Central Middlesex Hospital. Ruth's background in nursing and experience in collaborative care have supported her developing a whole systems approach to unifying elderly care provision in Brent. Her belief in user involvement and empowerment have provided significant learning through the presentation of problems from the user perspective.

Jean Andrews is from a Civil Service background. She spent 14 years briefing counsel to prosecute in the Crown Court. A further 5 years was spent in the Policy Division at Crown Prosecution Service headquarters, tackling a range of long-term, multi-agency projects. Jean's first contact with the NHS came as a project manager for the London Older People's Service Development Programme, setting up and developing a case finding project in Lambeth. Latterly, Jean has worked more closely with the Programme, offering help and support to the other project managers, particularly around co-ordinating services.

David Aron is Professor of Medicine and Epidemiology and Biostatistics at Case Western Reserve University and also Visiting Executive in Health Systems Management, Weatherhead School of Management, CWRU. Dr Aron received his MD at Columbia University College of Physicians and Surgeons and clinical training at the University of California, San Diego and University of California, San Francisco. He obtained the MS degree in Clinical Research Design and Statistical Analysis from the University of Michigan in 1995. He is Director of the Department of Veterans Affairs (VA) Quality Scholars Fellowship Program, a training program in quality improvement and Director of the Center for Quality Improvement Research. These two programs are located at the Louis Stokes Cleveland VA Medical Center where he serves as Associate Chief of Staff for Education.

Alan Beaton is project manager for Haringey Case Management Project, part of a two-year initiative through the London Older People's Service Development Programme. Seconded to Haringey

Teaching Primary Care NHS Trust from Barnet, Enfield and Haringey Mental Health NHS Trust, his background is Community Mental Health and still works as a Community Mental Health Nurse team leader for older people in Haringey.

Nigel Bell is Director of Service Transformation, in the Office of the e-Envoy, part of the Cabinet Office in the UK. He was the founding Chief Executive of the NHS Information Authority. Previous roles include global Director of Drug Development Information Systems (IS) at pharmaceuticals company Astra, European IS Director for an industrial group, management consultant with PriceWaterhouse, and several systems development positions. Nigel is a Chartered Engineer and Member of the British Computer Society, and has an (BSc) Hons degree in computer science and a masters (MSc) degree in managing change. He is a council member of the UK Partnership for Global Health.

Maxine Conner is the Director of the Learning Alliance, an NHS virtual team set up to support the service improvement and modernisation agenda in the north of England. Maxine designed and led the development of this successful organisation, which undertakes leading edge development work [see www.nyx.org.uk]. Maxine Conner has 20 years experience of improving health care delivery. She practised as a nurse, project manager and general manager within the NHS in both secondary and primary care. Her current area of practice is network development and she has a particular interest in organisation design, performance development and collaborative strategies for geographically distributed clinical networks.

Nigel Edwards is Director of Policy for the NHS Confederation, the membership organisation that represents 95% of Trusts and Health Authorities in the UK. His role is to influence health policy on behalf of member organisations and to help focus the dialogue with Government, the Department of Health and with other partner organisations. Prior to joining the NHS Confederation, Nigel ran London Health Economics Consortium, a research and consultancy company owned by the London School of Hygiene and Tropical Medicine and the University of York. His main interests there were in developing strategic plans for health economies and in research into new models of care delivery. Nigel is also a Visiting Professor at the London School of Hygiene and Tropical Medicine.

Sarah W. Fraser is well known in health care for her work on how good practice spreads, how improvements can be made at practitioner level and how organisations and teams can best work together. She is in demand as a speaker and workshop presenter, and has written numerous papers, articles and guides around the topics of spread, complexity, networks, collaboratives and improvements. As an independent consultant she spends much of her time working with large-scale improvement initiatives in the UK National Health Service. Her work also takes her to the USA, Canada, Sweden and other parts of Europe. She was employed for 10 years by Esso UK and held a variety of roles in the UK and in Europe, before joining the NHS in 1997. She is an honorary Visiting Professor at Middlesex University (London).

Stephen Guy is the Technology Manager for The Automation Partnership (TAP), suppliers of advanced automated systems, and has responsibility for formulating technology strategy for drug discovery, cell culture and genomics. He has forged a reputation for working on dynamic and interesting projects for organisations such as Formula One and the European Space Agency, and has unique experience of working on out-of-the-ordinary projects and pushing technology forward. He also has a great track record for forming and managing innovative and specialist teams of engineers.

Val Jones is Director, London Older People's Service Development Programme, seconded to the London Directorate of NHS Health and Social Care (previously London Region) for two years from Hammersmith and Fulham Social Services, where she held the post of Development Manager, Assessment and Rehabilitation. These two 'whole systems' posts have deepened her interest in partnership working and the development of coordinated services which promote a pro-active, preventative approach to older people's care.

Amanda Layton originally trained as a nurse and has worked in quality improvement since 1989. She began by researching the impact of medical audit within the medical profession, then moved to lead on the development of clinical protocols as part of the Patient Focused Project Team at Central Middlesex Hospital, London. She was Head of the Trust's Quality Department and led on the development of her Trust's strategy for Clinical Governance. In 1999 she became Project Director for West London for the first National Collaborative Programme on cancer service redesign. She is currently Head of the London Learning Partnership which provides a training and facilitation service for London in quality improvement techniques.

Penny Shuttleworth graduated from Durham University in History and then qualified as RGN at St Thomas' Hospital in 1985. She specialised in Occupational Health Nursing and won a Smith and Nephew Scholarship in 1991 to study Occupational Health Services in Barnaul, Siberia, developed IT and audit systems for Nottingham Occupational Health and completed an MBA in May 2001. She is currently working as a Workforce Designer for the Changing Workforce Programme, developing new roles around the care of Older People in North Derbyshire.

Helen Smith is currently Director of Workforce Development, North and East Yorkshire and Northern Lincolnshire Workforce Development Confederation. Before taking up this post in April 2002, she has undertaken a variety of roles in primary care, most recently as Primary Care Group Chief Executive in a very rural part of North Yorkshire. The organisation and development of primary care remains her greatest interest. Helen is married to a GP and has two sons.

Keith Strahan works in the London Borough of Hounslow as Project Manager for the Single Assessment Process. Keith previously was employed as the Primary Care Social Worker at Chiswick Health Centre in Hounslow where a feature of the casework was early intervention and direct allocation. Keith has also spent fifteen years as a Social Worker in inner London. Keith is committed to the development of 'person centred' care with older people and their carers and in a 'unified assessment process', which encourages good practice and joint working between health and social care agencies.

Dr Barry Tennison is currently Assistant Director for Policy and Development, and Public Health Advisor for the Commission for Health Improvement (CHI). Previously an academic mathematician, Barry trained as a doctor in his thirties and, after jobs in hospital medicine and surgery, psychiatry, geriatrics and general practice, specialised in Public Health Medicine, becoming a Consultant in 1989. Barry spent four years as Director of Information and Consultant in Public Health Medicine for Cambridge Health Authority, and Associate Lecturer at the Cambridge University Clinical School. He then moved in 1993 to

Hertfordshire as Director of Public Health for the newly formed Hertfordshire Health Agency. Following local reorganisation, from 1996 until 2000 he was Director of Public Health with West Hertfordshire Health Authority. He moved to CHI in July 2000, first to help develop the methods through which CHI reviews health authorities and primary care, and more lately with more general responsibilities for policy and development. He is also the public health advisor to CHI. Barry is an Honorary Professor in Public Health and Policy at the London School of Hygiene and Tropical Medicine.

Steve Unwin has over ten years experience of helping create organisational improvement. A former Head of Business Excellence for British Aerospace, winners of the UK Business Excellence Award, Steve recently founded Access to Excellence to promote the achievement of excellence in public and private sector organisations. Steve is a respected speaker on excellence issues and a regular conference and publication contributor. He played a key role supporting the EFQM development of the European Quality Model and is a prominent member of the UK Excellence Assessor Community. In a related project, he is near to completing 'The Explorer's Guide to Business Excellence' which explores the mind-set required for excellence. Steve is married with three children and is a keen supporter of Nottingham Forest Football Club.

Dr Tim Wilson has been a General Practitioner in south Oxfordshire in the UK for over ten years. In 1995, he became the youngest fellow of the Royal College of General Practitioners. His practice was one of the first to receive a Charter Mark from the Cabinet Office. Tim was a 2000/2001 Harkness Fellow working with Don Berwick to study quality improvement. In March 2000, Tim became Director of the RCGP Quality Unit which aims to support clinical governance leads in primary care. He has published articles regularly in the *BMJ*, *BJGP* and other journals and publications on poor performance, safety, presentation of information, and complexity. In 2002 he was awarded a Membership by distinction of the Faculty of Public Health Medicine. He is married with two children and enjoys working on his two allotments growing (occasionally) prize-winning vegetables.

David Yarrow has been practising, educating, researching and writing in the field of business improvement for 20 years. He began his working life in manufacturing industry, learning and applying approaches such as flexible manufacturing, just in time and theory of constraints. Since 1989, he has worked in Higher Education, running postgraduate courses in Quality Management and a range of programmes supporting the sharing of good practice across sectoral boundaries. Currently Head of the Centre for Business Excellence, at Newcastle Business School, UK, he is a firm believer that once we can develop the skill of lateral thinking and recognising 'generic' approaches for what they are, our ability to improve is greatly enhanced.

Foreword

People, the key ingredient

Steve Unwin

People make the difference

In creating this book we have sought to bring to health care a number of ideas under the heading of agility. The ideas have their roots in many different areas; different worlds that have devised ways of dealing with situations and circumstances. We have sought in particular to capture some of the experience from the world of manufacturing and production, a world where people make things, in the belief that they have value in the world of health care. Our aim is to identify how learning from the first may be transferred to the second of these worlds. This is not to say in any way that the world of production is superior to the world of health care; indeed the opportunity for the flow of learning is in both directions. Each world has developed skills and knowledge in particular areas by virtue of the focus of attention on the particular tasks it performs. The accident of circumstance has created the need and driven the development of a number of techniques in the production world that we feel may be of value.

The world of production has achieved some degree of success in adopting change and adapting its processes to meet changing demand. This ability to change and better satisfy the needs of stakeholders is central to what we wish to share and is central to the idea of agility. In a changing world, and few would attempt to argue that the pace of change is other than increasing, that ability to adapt to changing needs has become critical to the success or even the survival of many businesses. This requirement to change constantly, to be able to identify new needs of clients and customers, is not a passing business fad. It is driven by those customers and clients seeking and demanding more for their money year on year and day by day. I and you, the reader, are part of this demand. Whilst we may think that we hanker after traditional values and the old ways, if we were to be offered many of the products produced even thirty or so years ago we would fall about laughing.

You're not convinced? Well my first car was a Vauxhall Viva HB Deluxe built in the late 1960s. By the time I got it, it was past its prime, but when new had looked a treat in the showroom window and was a car many aspired to own at the time. My Viva was in a colour that I chose to call British Racing Green, which I'm sure made it that little bit faster. Mine was no standard model. Mine was the DeLuxe. It earned the grand title of DeLuxe not because it had passenger airbags, satellite navigation or central locking, these were many years in the future, nor because it had power assisted steering, electric windows or even leather seats, for it had none of these, though it did have a windscreen water squirter that worked by pushing a plunger on the dashboard. No it earned the title DeLuxe because it had a heater fitted as standard. Can you imagine anyone buying a car today that didn't have a heater? Today's cars have so many built in features that if the boot were decorated with badges proclaiming them, in the style of the sixties, there wouldn't be any space for the number-plate!

Our exposure to what can be achieved, either through excellent products or exceptional service ensures that our sights are constantly set higher, and our tolerance of poor performance, products or service, in whatever form, grows lower. Here poor performance encompasses not just those organisations that have grown worse, but also those that have failed to grow better quickly enough to keep pace with expectations.

As we know our demands for better performance are not confined to private sector companies. We demand more of public sector organisations and indeed even of 'not for profit' organisations. If we are giving a pound to charity we want to see absolutely as much as possible going where it was intended and not consumed in management or administration costs. And we all have higher expectations than we used to of the way that our taxes will be spent on the provision of public services.

In setting out to create the book, we have gathered a broad range of contributors, each with specialist knowledge, ideas and perspectives, with the aim of creating a rich picture of opportunities to benefit from the available learning. If you read through the book you will see these different contributions, some describing tools, processes or approaches, whilst others use models to convey ideas, each drawn from their wide experience.

We, the contributors to this book, come from wide and varied backgrounds. Whilst we each knew some of the others before we embarked on this project we have all made new friends. As we began to pull together our ideas, often little more than scribbled notes or vaguely drawn notions at the outset, we started to share our past experience. We could each feel a common thread, a theme which linked all of our thoughts. Whilst each was bringing different models, tools and techniques, and sharing our different successes and failures, we each carried a common belief. Our shared belief is not a profound one, but it is a critical one. The tools, techniques and models are important but they are minor and often incidental players in the act of creating change. Centre stage is of course reserved for the people within the organisation. People are the key to achieving change, and it is through people, their attitudes and approaches, that tools stand or fall.

As a reader of this book, you declare an interest in creating change. Already by selecting to read this text you are a rarity, what we might term a scarce resource. At the most simple level, our aim to help enable change in health care, is channelled through you, the reader. We invite you to centre stage and the glare of the spotlight. We know it feels a little uncomfortable, to be singled out on your own, with everyone watching and waiting to hear what you have to say or see what you plan to do. This book is about helping you take on the challenge of change and to succeed.

Our joint and collective experience is that if people aren't ready for change, it won't take place. This is true for production and is true for health care. Now you are the first link in our chain of communicating between the two worlds. In creating change in health care you are key. In this short chapter we hope to begin to help you consider your attitude to change, so before we take a look at some of the changes in manufacturing let's just check if you are open to learning.

Can we transfer learning between these worlds?

If your only experience of a production environment was a school metalwork class sometime in the dim and distant past, modern production facilities would come as something of a surprise. Whilst there are still companies that would have a recognisable feel, a modern car plant would strike you as positively space age. Thousands of employee operations have been replaced by robots often operating with uncanny human like dexterity and deftness as they manoeuvre large assemblies into position with unerring precision.

Though different to the past there is no doubt that a production environment looks, feels, sounds and even smells different to a hospital or health centre. The products of these two environments are different, and so are the tools and techniques used to produce them, so does this mean that they can't learn from each other? Well that may be an understandable initial reaction, to see the differences, to identify the things that characterise one environment and are absent from the other and reason that they provide the proof that learning cannot be transferred.

This problem is not just a feature when trying to move between the worlds. Within the world of production, there are many organisations and people who concentrate on seeing the differences. The truth is that the ideas that we are about to explain have yet to be adopted by many manufacturing companies. And the single most frequent reason given is that the organisation in question is 'different'. Its products are bigger or smaller, more complex or simpler, use different materials, are produced in different places or have different designs and each of these differences stands in the way of learning. Much like the football supporter who only sees that you wear blue whilst he wears red, these organisations only see the differences and these differences are used to excuse the need to learn.

The reality is that those organisations that have benefited from these ideas are as diverse as those that have not. There is no common factor in their products or service, their location or the materials they use that ties them together. They are instead tied by their thinking and approach, and by their willingness to transfer and apply learning. Those that look beyond the differences are the ones who stand to benefit.

But the pressure to resist learning can be strong, a feeling that you are different and therefore cannot learn and benefit. This is an understandable but mistaken belief – reject it. We are all unique, we are all different and in a changing world we aren't simply different to each other, we are different to ourselves day by day. This is what continuous improvement is; a continuously changing definition of ourselves and our environment. We are all different, but we are all facing the challenge of change. That's what we share and that's what makes us the same.

What we aim to share through this book is not focussed in the realms of what to do, but on this experience of dealing with the need to change, of becoming adept at anticipating, implementing and succeeding in change.

Whilst we are looking at reasons often given not to change, a second reason to avoid learning stems from a feeling of inferiority, that you know so little of a subject that it impossible to make up ground. This is equally mistaken. We have confessed that there are many in the production world that would benefit from the understanding that you are about to gain. But more than this, one of the lessons we have learned is that learning is only achieved when there is a sharing of ideas and there is much that production people can and will need to learn from the health care sector.

Well now we've considered and hopefully removed, some of the obstacles to learning, let's move on.

Our aim is to help facilitate the transfer of some of the knowledge and experience gained in the production world into the world of health care. It is not, however, our intention to tell you what to do. We don't believe we could do that. We recognise that those involved in health care grapple with its issues, its problems and challenges every day. It would be more than a little presumptuous and unwise to claim that we have the answers, but more important it would run counter to our interest in creating agility.

As you read through this volume you will discover the topic of agility viewed from a number of perspectives with different contributors bringing different facets into perspective. For the moment it is enough to understand that agility is the ability to sense, to interpret, to plan and to act to create changes that allow your organisation to better meet the changing demands placed upon it. And to do this in the certain knowledge that whatever solution you arrive at will be overtaken by newer and newer solutions as you respond to an ever-changing environment and address ever-changing needs.

Agility isn't about having the answer. It's about having the ability to repeatedly refresh, update and amend your answer, and to relish the challenge of doing so. We set out, not to provide our view of the answer, but to share our experience of how some organisations have arrived at some of their answers and how these helped them to move on.

Note that these answers themselves are part of an ongoing renewal process and they will each be replaced as organisations progress. It is terribly tempting to rubbish an answer once it has reached the point of being replaced. Avoid this thinking. It is the death of continuous improvement. Agile organisations are those that move to replace ways of working when required to meet need. They don't hang on to them long after their sell by date, nor replace them with the latest initiative for the sake of fashion. As an envoy of agility you will need to learn that it is the fate of all ideas, however brilliant, at the appropriate time to pass into history, and their passing is neither to be mourned nor ridiculed, but recognised for the contribution it made. Even my Vauxhall Viva HB Deluxe has its little entry in the history of the motor car and without it we wouldn't have reached the point we have.

So we don't intend to provide answers, but we do plan to share knowledge which we hope will spark your thinking; to serve up some ideas and, we hope, stimulate you to find your answers, and keep finding them. And remember this should not be a solitary activity. Whilst you may feel alone in your spotlight, there are others feeling equally exposed. Within their spotlight in other areas of the health care world and within the production world and a whole host of other worlds they are all grappling with the same problems, wrapped up in different packaging.

Sharing ideas

The production world has the benefit of many years of development of ideas and approaches to dealing with the processes of bringing together resources, capabilities and requirements to produce what the customer wants, when the customer wants it, quickly, smoothly and efficiently. This learning has not been gained without a fair number of stumbles and grazed knees, not to mention some rather more dramatic and public disasters. This hard won learning has been bought at considerable cost. This gives us considerable confidence that there is some powerful raw material with which to share; a good starting point!

When we think of learning from others, it is useful to separate the learning into two categories. First there is the learning of the skills and techniques, the expertise perhaps honed through years of practice. The second element of learning is how these skills were developed, how was the need identified, how were the skills defined, improved and built upon, how was their effectiveness evaluated and reviewed. We think of these two quite different elements of learning because each holds different value for us as we try to learn.

Perhaps an example might help. Let us imagine that I have the opportunity to listen to the experience of an Olympic athlete. Any athlete would do. It could be an Olympic weight lifter or ice skater for example. Now I may not have met you, the reader, but if I had, following even the most fleeting of encounters you would readily conclude that the techniques of weight lifting are not a subject of special interest to me. I would find little if any value in having revealed to me the intricacies of the 'clean and jerk'. Equally the figure skating champion need not fear that I wish to steal the secret of the triple-salko. What I am sure I could learn from each of these champions are the ways in which they became champions. Whilst this may touch upon the skills of their chosen sport, the focus would be on 'hows', not 'whats'. How did they decide on their goals? How did they identify appropriate performance measures and comparisons? How did they focus their work? How did they deal with disappointment and set back? How did they identify which were the key skills they needed to perfect? These and a thousand other questions would be of direct relevance to me in my quest to become better and be the best at whatever is my chosen field. Indeed, should the champions stray into the details of their sport, I may redirect them back to the topic of becoming a champion, rather than describing how to lift 200 kilos or pirouette across a sheet of ice, however incredible and impossible these feats may appear to me.

Willingness to question, to challenge and to adopt learning is the fundamental prerequisite for achieving change. Before reaching that point it is so easy to find the reasons to not change pervading and undermining thinking.

For example:

Have you ever had a flat tyre? How long did it take to change? Perhaps around 20 minutes. Who would believe that all four tyres could be changed in 7 seconds? But, as Formula One enthusiasts see at every race, this feat has become so routine that to take 15 seconds is considered a disaster.

Have you ever put up a shelf? How long did that take? Thirty minutes might be impressive. How about building a ship? Think it could be done in a month? The Liberty Ships were wartime transport ships used to transport materials and equipment from America to Europe. They were over four hundred feet long and could transport over 9,000 tons of cargo. These were significant pieces of engineering! At the start of production, the first ships took 225 to 230 days. Once production had got into full swing the shortest time taken to produce one was the Robert G Peary which took an astonishing 4 days 15 hours and 30 minutes from laying down the keel to launch! It was fitted out and ready for sea and its maiden voyage three days later.

In the world of production, the advances made, such as they are, were made in environments where, before they were achieved, they appeared impossible, indeed they were impossible. They were achieved by looking at a problem as a challenge to be overcome. In each case the solution has its roots in the problem. No Formula One team could contemplate a race in which a tyre change would take 20 minutes. The need drove the desire and identification of a solution. By the same token, the need to feed and re-supply Europe during the Second World War meant that literally thousands of ships would need to be built, not over a ten-year period, but in a matter of months. Between 1939 and 1945, over five thousand US Liberty Ships were ordered. This was five times the 1939 total national fleet of the US.

The quick wheel change and the Liberty Ship each provide examples of how a range of techniques have been brought together to achieve the seemingly impossible. Some of the techniques are technical. The liberty ships used mass production techniques where major components were pre-assembled before being brought together. Special tools are sometimes used. For example, the Formula One approach replaces the wheel nuts with which we are familiar with a quick-fit attachment. Each example also demonstrates the importance of team-working. We see this in a flash during a race pit stop, but imagine the teamwork required to manage the hundreds of people and thousands of tons of steel and equipment that has to be arranged to be in just the right place at just the right time to build a liberty ship in four days. Each example ably demonstrates that, in reality, achieving the magic of seemingly impossible performance requires a blend of approaches of people, technology, tools, techniques and methods. The answer seldom lies in one change, but in a coordinated suite of changes.

Maybe you knew all about tyre changes in seven seconds and they don't impress any more, but building a ship in less than a week? Perhaps you are thinking that of course shipyards are different, or maybe in war time it's different, or maybe in the US it's different, or any of a thousand other differences you could choose to see.

Remember the impossible is only impossible because it's never been done. Once the 'impossible' has been mastered it soon becomes the 'routine'. These previous impossibilities are all around us, and we soon rely on them to live our routine lives.

Agile organisations are always ready to question, to challenge, to change and to do it all over again and again. The starting point for all change is people being prepared to accept that change can be achieved.

Are you?

1 | Introduction to agility

Sarah W. Fraser, David J. Yarrow, Maxine Conner

One of the paradoxes we face in health care is an instinctive pull towards treating each patient and service user as unique, as opposed to the need to 'standardise' some parts of the patients journey as part of a drive to improve services. Is health care following in the footsteps of industry's experiences of the 1990s by driving itself towards 'mass customisation', compromising individuals' unique needs because of the difficulties they pose, even though we are in an era when personalisation is the hallmark?

Change is not something that comes along when someone has a good idea for a project or restructuring. It happens every day and involves everyone. One certainty is that the pace of change will continue to accelerate. Health care is no different to other industries in feeling the implications of the new knowledge economy with its explosion of information and focus on the power of tacit and explicit knowledge. Combine this with growing patient and consumer expectations of services and the challenges become obvious – more change, more quickly.

Health care has traditionally borrowed change methodologies from the private sector. This is not surprising as the more innovative and less risk-averse companies, with profit as a driver, have the incentive to invest the resources necessary to test and develop new ways of implementing change. This means the public sector is often 5 to 10 years behind the private sector in using their tried and tested methods. For example, business process re-engineering was an early 1990s phenomenon in industry, and the National Health Service (NHS) is currently using it as a prime method of change, renaming it redesign.[i] Some NHS organisations have developed approaches to redesign that build upon truly 'bottom up' approach and focus upon a wide range of results to ensure effectiveness of the change effort.[ii]

The public sector has some fundamental and obvious differences from the private sector; namely it is about *people*, delivering *people-based* services, using (predominantly) the taxpayers' money. In contrast, whilst some of the private sector, such as service

[i] Locock L, *Maps and Journeys: Redesign in the NHS.* The University of Birmingham Health Services Management Centre, 2001.

[ii] Stahr H, Bulman B, Stead M, *The Excellence Model in Healthcare,* Chichester, Kingsham Press, UK, 2000.

[iii] Womack JP, Jones DT, *Lean Thinking; Banish Waste and Create Wealth in your Corporation*. Simon & Schuster, New York, 1996.

[iv] Monden Y, *Toyota Production System: Practical Application to Production Management*. Industrial Engineering and Management Press, Georgia, 1983.

[v] Goldratt E, 'Focusing on constraints, not costs'. In *Rethinking the Future*, edited by Gibson R, Nicholas Brierly Publishing, London, 1998.

[vi] Department of Health, *The NHS Plan: a Plan for Investment : a Plan for Reform*, HMSO, July, 2000.

industries, also has a similar people-based context, industry is mainly concerned with the production of goods to sell to customers, for a profit. It is from these production industries, due to their pursuit of reduced costs and improved quality, and the tangibility of their materials, their products and their waste, that the majority of change and improvement methodologies have emerged.

One such approach is 'lean thinking'.[iii] This originated as a means of reducing the waste generated in production processes by focusing on what adds value. It is also characterised by pulling items through the chain of production and supply, rather than pushing, and by efforts to understand and optimise the entire supply chain, rather than focusing only on its constituent parts, as well as the desire to recognise and manage constraints. This can lead to substantial improvements in the speed of flow through the system. And the flow isn't just faster, it's also better in many other ways – smoother, more reliable, more visible, less costly, more readily improvable.[iv,v]

Improving the speed, and the consistency, at which patients are seen is one of the UK government's highest priorities for health care,[vi] so it is no surprise to see lean thinking starting to take over from business process redesign as a change methodology in the NHS. The future of organisations and service providers will depend upon their ability to apply the most appropriate improvement methodologies to the task they face. Organisations and leaders must have at their fingertips a range of methodologies if they are to be truly agile – delivering excellent quality care by continuously developing and co-evolving with changing demands and requirements. The current situation is one in which organisations appear to flounder from one fad to another. Organisations need to have wide-ranging competence, maintain it and deploy it wisely. The people within organisations need to learn about a variety of improvement approaches, understanding how to diagnose the underlying context and apply them appropriately will be a feature of those mastering the improvement agenda. This is part of the strategy to 'manage' capacity and demand whilst delivering service level change.

Laudable stuff. But what happens to the people in all this? Lean thinking uses a language that betrays its manufacturing origins. Some patient processes can be likened to production lines, making it more apparent that the concepts might be applicable. Techniques such as 'KanBan', which involves the next work station signalling 'I'm ready' before the previous stage sends it a new product to work on, might be adapted to assist a patient process to switch its emphasis from 'push' to 'pull'. Setting up reduction and preventative maintenance schemes are as important in the operating theatre as they are on the factory shop floor. And while 'eliminating buffer stocks' might not sound too friendly, it doesn't take much lateral thinking to see the parallels with patient delays half way through a process.

There is nothing wrong with lean thinking or many other production-orientated methodologies. Indeed there is much the NHS can learn and gain insight to help improve its own services. The danger is trying to take methodologies and applying them wholesale, without testing and adapting them first. There is a high probability that they won't work at first, and a risk that by the time we make them work, it will be too late. Good ideas, with lots of potential to help us, can be discredited before they get a chance to prove their worth. The trial and adaptation phase is crucial. One of the useful experiences of business process re-engineering (BPR) was the use of pilot sites that helped create new terms and descriptions more applicable to the NHS and to identify which pieces tended not to work. For example, the redesign work done at Leicester Royal Infirmary in the mid-1990s was significant in creating the NHS language about BPR and also identified the difficulty in working with core processes such as human resources, finances, research and development.

Our health care 'production lines' are composed of human beings (both the patients and the staff) who operate freely and interact with one another in a way that is not as linear as the experience of the production line. By the same token, not all factories contain neat, linear flow-lines making identical products in their hundreds and thousands. There is much to learn too from the jobbing shop and the fabrication yard, whose production systems owe as much to project management techniques as to *Just in Time* regularity and flow. However, even production-orientated industries that lend themselves readily to BPR and lean thinking are realising the shortfalls; the time it takes to make the changes, the limited ability to keep adapting to the changing environment and customers' expectations (and thus limited sustainability of results), and the potentially negative impact on staff. Perhaps the greatest danger encountered by many industries and companies is the curse of 'Initiative-Overload'. Each shiny new management technique looks so appealing sitting there on the shelf, or in the management consultant's brochure, just waiting to be plugged into your company. But a poorly implemented solution can be not only disappointing, but also counter-productive. Perhaps it was the right solution for the wrong problem? All too often the response has been to move swiftly on to the next 'magic bullet'. 'The last one didn't work' is the cry. A wiser head might conclude that 'we didn't make it work … and there's a good chance that the pattern will repeat'.

So where does this leave improvement initiatives in health care? Rather than picking up old change methods, why not test out some of the more innovative approaches being implemented by those industries that believe the future lies in delivering the customer's personal needs and not in the mass customisation 'fit your needs to this solution' approach – industries where the emphasis is on developing the capability to adapt to continuous change, rather than the delivery and implementation of designed solutions. For example, the motor manufacturing industry is now focusing on how to deliver a car in three days, with exactly the customised specification required by the customer.

The philosophy that treats each customer as unique, leverages its resources through applying various improvement methods and focuses on the ability of production lines and employees to continually adapt and co-evolve with changing conditions, is called *'Agility'*. Developed in the USA and adopted by leading edge companies worldwide, agile systems aim to respond to rapidly changing and fragmented environments and market places. Through flexible working, long-term relationships with suppliers and partners, including the customer, a focus on co-operation and virtual teaming, improvements wider than just speed are delivered. They include cost, service and quality. This is not a touchy-feely philosophy. It is underpinned by tough 'lean thinking' type principles to reduce waste, improve flow and optimise results.

The attractiveness of this methodology is twofold: its ability to bring the people dimension into the change process and the focus on design that is flexible, adaptable and consequently sustainable over the longer term.

Another methodology, another piece of rhetoric? Possibly. However, there are already teams testing out how the concepts apply in the NHS and how improvement can be leveraged through a combination of production line thinking and people-orientated empathy. And there are already many examples of 'agility' in practice in the NHS, mostly unrecognised as such and perhaps under-exploited in terms of the benefits they could be delivering. The most fertile ground for this is in community, primary, social and mental health care, where the uniqueness of the patient or service user is a key focus. They are focusing on delivering improvements in radical and flexible forms, through involving a wide number of stakeholders, and with an eye on continual adaptability to enable long-term sustainability. Their remit is a challenging one – to improve their services, become leading edge examples of agility in action, and to do all this without a high profile. The fear is that raising the profile will launch 'Agility' as yet another untested methodology for a tools and technique-weary NHS. Time, and results, will demonstrate the extent to which 'Agility' is a useful model for the health sector.

Agility, an additional philosophy for those who see their patients as unique, their organisation as a co-evolving and flexible group of teams, and their staff as significant contributing factors for the sustainability of improved services.

Overview of the chapters in this 'Reader' on Agility

The foreword, **People, the key ingredient**, as the name suggests, reminds us that in the midst of a plethora of tools, techniques and concepts, it is the people in the system, and the people designing and changing the systems, who will determine the degree of success or failure. People are the key to achieving improvement, and it is through people, their attitudes and approaches, that tools stand or fail.

Thriving in unpredictable times sets the scene by surfacing the key issues that suggest linear production line thinking is insufficient a methodology for the ever shifting business of health care. The authors use the concepts of adaptive systems to challenge the notion of 'sustainability' and list some principles for how not just to survive but also how to make the most of unpredictable situations.

Lean processes are the foundation of agile systems and in the chapter **Planning and scheduling; maintaining flow in adaptive systems**, the authors set the scene and challenges for health care processes. They introduce three levels of health care scheduling systems; level one is basic, level two lean and level three agile – each level with more demanding requirements and increasing efficiency and client satisfaction. **Reducing work in progress and waste** continues on from the previous chapter and looks in detail at the concept of *pulling* the patient through the systems, instead of *pushing*.

One of the key tools and techniques for understanding and improving processes is the use of process mapping. However, in unpredictable systems this technique can be supplemented with a higher-level approach which enables the surfacing of the system, in all its mess and complexity. **Using stock, flow and trigger (SiFT) mapping to visualise, analyse and improve systems** is a chapter which provides you with an overview of a new technique based on systems dynamics modelling combined with the push/pull concept from production engineering.

Systems need excellent supporting structures and in **Maximising the use of information systems** Nigel Bell sets out the challenge for information management and technology in supporting agile health care systems. This includes the role of knowledge management and customer relationship management in helping systems listen to the outside; the challenges of exploiting enterprise resource planning systems in order to utilise all of an organisation's resources; the potential for decision support systems and the promise of intelligent software agents for maintaining responsiveness; and the use of extranets and information standards to extend an organisation's capabilities.

This book then shifts from the technical to the people factors. Maxine Conner presents the case for **Teaming and leading in agile systems**. Agile teams can be recognised by their responsiveness and adaptability as well as their ability to anticipate changes and new requirements. Leading these types of teams requires a breadth of vision and practicality of operation. The chapter ends with some simple ways in which the concepts can be put into action in your local health care community.

So where is some of this happening? In **The journey to agility; case studies from improving the care for older adults in London** the authors share their emerging stories about how they are working in ways to develop agile services. These are early examples and ones designed to provide you with a feel for what might be accomplished, as well as the practicalities of doing so. They are, of course, still developing and improving!

Developing agile primary care organisations; using network principles as the basis for organisational design investigates how organisational design needs to be considered if agile systems are to be a reality. Using the principles of networks, the authors suggest that size of team, connectivity and purpose are all keys for creating agile systems.

Performance management is difficult and is often a contested management process in very ordinary and stable times. However, when the environment is unpredictable and organisations and services are going through major changes, the challenge is increased. In **Performance managing agile organisations** Barry Tennison and David Yarrow provide a framework to structure your thinking. They investigate the concept of measurement and the use of performance indicators. Is the issue one of performance management or performance development – they'll let you be the judge of that.

Agile systems need also to be safer systems. In **Coping with uncommon calamities; building safer systems**, David Aron describes organisational vulnerability and the inevitability of calamity. Some organisations have found ways to survive this inevitability through preventative and responsive actions and in this chapter there are some examples and ideas on how to ensure your health care system is a safer one.

Agility as a concept is not just applicable to health care services; it is also applicable to other areas such as the development of drugs. In **Personalised therapeutics impact on treatment efficiency** Stephen Guy provides an overview as to how agile systems can focus on the benefit to the individual.

So what? The final chapter of this reader looks at the **Policy implications** of agile systems. Within the context of the UK, the authors discuss *how* policy can inhibit agility through its ideology and processes. The implications of developing policy in a way to enable agility are substantial, though not impossible.

2 | Thriving in unpredictable times

Tim Wilson, Barry Tennison, Sarah W. Fraser

Introduction

Health care throughout the world is faced with increasing quality problems. Advances in medical technology increase expectations daily, but what people want is far more than treatment options and cures. The public and patients rightly demand a high standard of service that matches their needs and values. The health care system cannot simply provide a single process that suits all patients. Not only will that process be out of date very rapidly but it does not recognise that each person's experience of care is a personal issue, affected by their beliefs, perceptions and context. Mass customisation goes some way towards this; however, it cannot hope to meet the needs of everyone. What is needed is an agile system – one that is lean, flexible and adaptable.

This chapter highlights the ever-changing environment within which health care is delivered and suggests that organisations and processes that meet, and continue to meet, patient and stakeholder expectations, are flexible and continually transforming. They are systems that are sensitive to external shifts and where non-permanent teams merge and reform around individual needs.

The limitations of traditional thinking

Refining crude oil is a complex and at times dangerous process. Refineries are very complicated structures with many sub-systems and connections between units and pipelines. There are intricate control systems linked to a command centre staffed by a few managers, engineers and technicians where most activities can be

Acknowledgement
Some of the material for this chapter has previously been published in Fraser SW, 2001, 'Adapting to improvement', Health Management. Reused with permission from the Institute of Health Care Management.

carried out by remote control; for example, opening or closing a valve. An alarm will sound when something goes wrong and staff can refer to manuals to find out where the problem is and how they can fix it. Whilst this is going on, production is usually reduced or stopped.

Although hospital and primary care practices are also complex with interlinking processes, they are substantially different from refineries and other production systems. Yet many of the improvement methodologies being applied in health care, particularly in the US and Europe, such as business process reengineering, come from these production models. In addition, quality and customer service models have been borrowed from sectors such as banking and the airline industry. Whilst some improvement may be achieved by using these techniques, there are often difficulties in implementing and sustaining system-wide improvements using such methods, particularly the production-orientated ones.

The main reason for this is that health care is a behavioural system; the processes and products of any system like health care are significantly dependent on individuals and the way they behave. In a refinery, valves don't open and close of their own accord – in health care, practitioners and managers will act in ways that reflect their personal motivations, the circumstances of their role and their personal professional judgement. These sorts of systems, where independent agents act in ways that impact upon other independent agents, are called 'complex adaptive systems' (see Box 1).

They are *complex* because just one small change by one person can have a large impact on the whole of the system, without there being the possibility of predicting what might happen. Alternatively, the converse is often seen, where large-scale changes have little impact.

Change is not linear. It often happens spontaneously out of a disorganised or apparently destructive or tense situation. This can result in new and innovative ways of working.

Behavioural systems are *adaptive* because the individuals in them can make decisions about what to do and can change the course of events. They can change themselves in ways that a pipe or valve can't. This also means they can also resist change in ways that a valve or pipe can't! Empirical observation suggests that, in response to external pressure or change, a behavioural system adapts in a way that tends to resist change. It is this non-linearity, adaptability and lack of predictability, which is one of the main reasons why health care is difficult to organise, both strategically and operationally. Add to this the wide variety of types of care, the

Box 1: Complex adaptive systems (CAS)

These are systems which are usually composed of numerous, relatively independent elements which:

- interact with each other in non-linear ways, often with each element interacting most with only a few other ('local') elements
- are not subject to an overall mechanistic control
- interact with their environment in open ways, with exchange of things like energy and/or information

They often exhibit

- *self-organisation*; that is, without a set of detailed instructions they produce an ordered pattern of behaviour
- *emergence*; that is, the patterns of behaviour that evolves is often unpredictable and is completely novel, often producing something more effective than before
- *adaptation and evolution,* with the whole system appearing to change, often *co-evolving* with other complex adaptive systems

Examples might be:

- the global weather system, whose elements are the molecules of the atmosphere: self-organises into weather systems, where emergent phenomena include fronts and storms
- national political systems, with self-organisation into parties and coalitions and emergent phenomena like consensus views and policies
- many biological systems, including the body of any animal; a single species; or a local ecosystem
- a national economy, with self-organisation into companies and industries, and emergent properties like interest rates
- a single health care provider organisation, perhaps a group of hospitals, with the staff and professional groups interacting with patients and the local community
- a 'health community' consisting of a population and all the people and organisations that provide them with health care
- a national health system, with many interacting parts, and emergent policies and practices, evolving over time.

[i] Sackett D, Haynes B, Tugwell P, Guyatt G, *Clinical Epidemiology: A Basic Science for Clinical Medicine.* Hagerstown, MD USA. Lippincott Williams & Wilkins Publishers, 1991.

[ii] Freeman AC, Sweeney K, Why general practitioners do not implement evidence: qualitative study, *BMJ;* 323: 1100, 2001.

different professions, organisations and teams that all have their own operating standards, and then the different agendas set by patients, carers and their network of families, friends and other input (e.g. the media) – the challenges become obvious…

Unpredictability

It is very hard to predict what happens in health care (see Box 2). This is an important issue, given that patients are *dis-eased,* and the health care system should help alleviate their suffering. It is uncertain how or what should be done. Who is best placed to provide the care, what system is best to deliver the care, what formulary should be used locally? Although research can tell us that at a macro or population level, one action is broadly better than another in controlled circumstances, as soon as other 'complicating' factors are taken into consideration, detailed and dynamic complexity comes into play.[i] What might be predictable in the context of a randomised controlled trial is often unpredictable in the context of daily, person, patient care. This has been one of the major criticisms of the evidence-based movement, which although providing the highest quality information for clinicians, has yet to see its impact in daily care. Whilst it is difficult to know why this might be, it is likely that the mismatch between the evidence and the person in front of the clinician is a large factor – the evidence is simple, the patient more complex.[ii]

However, although this is true, evidence-based medicine (EBM) does provide a guide as to what can be achieved. Just as the weather is boundable (it is colder in January than in July) but not predictable (not every day in July will be warmer than every day in January), so is patient care. Whilst taking aspirin after a heart attack reduces the risk of future coronary events, a system cannot be designed simply to deliver aspirin to all suitable people. Some will have had previous problems with aspirin, not just obvious contraindications to taking it, but perhaps other events that affect their judgement. Further, they may have read something about taking aspirin or had a friend or relative with problems with aspirin. Many people may not like to be medicalised by taking aspirin every day. Lastly, it is impossible to state whether taking aspirin will prevent a further coronary event in this patient. Although on the basis of trial data it will reduce the risk, it is impossible to predict exactly what will happen. Taking all these into consideration means that health care is, even with a simple problem, unpredictable and uncertain.

Box 2: Changes in the world of medicine

Medication – although some drugs are less suitable for certain ethnic groups it is generally impossible to predict whether a patient will respond well to a specific medication or whether they will get what is termed a predictable (that is common) side effect or an idiosyncratic reaction. In truth it is impossible to predict what effect the medicine will have.

Concordance – some patients will blithely accept any medication their doctor prescribes whilst others will refuse outright. The majority are somewhere in the middle – sometimes taking the medication, sometimes not and generally dosing themselves in an unpredictable way ('oh, I feel better today, I'll leave them off'). This constant variation in medication dosing means that prediction is again impossible; for example, taking a blood pressure tablet when a patient is about to see the doctor will likely lower the recorded blood pressure reading in the surgery but not for the rest of the time.

Guidelines – these sometimes have a major impact on the behaviour of the health care system. In retrospect it can be easy to determine why (it was printed on coloured paper, it matched current changes in practice). But usually their impact is far from predictable and generally minimal.

Why control and rigid procedures and protocols make things worse

Complex adaptive systems are self-organising and appear to reflect an inherent sense of control and order, without there being a central command centre. Think of all the changes the NHS has undergone in the last 52 plus years – despite what many will think about the perceived chaos and disruption, patients have continued to be cared for and services delivered. Moreover, health professionals are highly educated and valued for the *discretion* they bring to caring for patients. Their patients would not want them to be following blindly a set of precise rules, but rather to be taking into account all the manifold individual circumstances of each patient, and using their judgement to advise and treat *that individual* for the best.

iii Mullan F, A Founder Of Quality Assessment Encounters A Troubled System Firsthand. Shortly before his death, Avedis Donabedian talked with about health care and the management of his own cancer care. *Health Affairs*, 20(1); 137–142, 2001.

iv Berwick D, 'Run to space' Address to the National Forum for Health care Improvement Dec 6, 1995.

Rigid control can also have untoward effects in other way. It is possible that the instructions that have to be followed might easily contradict local values (e.g. all patients who cannot speak English must have a translator – it may be felt, by patient and clinician that imposition of a translator destroys the clinician–patient relationship). This very contradiction might lead to 'rebellious' action or 'resistance to change' when local innovation would perhaps have come up with other more suitable solutions. Furthermore, focussing on specific priorities means that other, perhaps more important, issues are ignored. For example, the imposition of a national policy that in vitro fertilisation (IVF) should be publicly funded would probably divert funds away from other local priorities, perhaps in maternity or other services. The responses to disasters, like the Ronan Point building collapse (expensive tightening of building regulations) or the deaths of several schoolchildren on an organised canoeing trip (legislation to register certain types of leisure providers) were arguably disproportionate in the costs, financial and effort that they imposed. Last, in order to achieve goals or targets set, pointless activities are instigated to 'massage' the figures when other activities, based around higher-level concepts, might be more appropriate.

The use of performance measurement within health care can act as a deterrent to evolution and innovation. Whilst it is right and proper that patients should expect to know the quality of care they receive, use of external measurement, such as monitoring adherence to guidelines and policies does not always capture this. Avedis Donabedian clearly stated that what patients value most is a caring health care system.[iii] Don Berwick highlighted that it is sometimes impossible to measure care.[iv]

A rigid system designed to perform in one particular manner (for example, record and act on preventive problems) will not be able to provide the same type of care to an unemployed drug addict with HIV and an elderly war veteran with diabetes. Both may have their weight and blood pressure taken, be given smoking advice and advised on a healthy diet (all regularly measured as aspects of quality) but will this be what they want and need? The war veteran might want to continue smoking, as it is the only pleasure in his life, whilst the drug addict might be most concerned about starting a family with his partner.

Thriving; redefining sustainability

If predicting the nature of health care in detail is impossible then what kind of model is needed to ensure services cope with these issues?

First, *how* will health care survive? Much is made of achieving specific goals or targets in health care and then holding the gains; that is once you are there, stay there. If something appears to be good then why not do it? There are many reasons why not; it may not be in keeping with what the patient needs, what the patient wants and very soon may not be the best method or process due to changes in health care technology.

Secondly, people change, patients change, the environment changes and technology changes. Some of these changes are large and important, reversing current ideas, other are subtler. However, as we have described, the more subtle changes may have more lasting or profound effects due to the non-linear way in which change occurs in a complex adaptive system. Further, teams of health care workers keep changing as new skills and experiences constantly alter the content and nature of the service they can deliver. Success is more that just holding the gains it is about co-evolving to meet new needs and to respond to new circumstances.

Sustainability, therefore, means meeting what lies ahead and not what is happening now. Planning to overcome a current crisis is important but building solutions for the next crisis before it happens is far better. It is not possible to predict what these problems might be, therefore a system that thrives and survives will build capability (see Figure 1). Highly reliable organisations

v Stephenson J, 'Capability and quality in higher education' in Stephenson J, York M, eds. *Capability and Quality in Higher Education*, Kogan-Page, London, 1995.

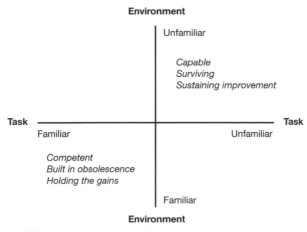

Stephenson, 1995

Figure 1[v]

vi Bristol Inquiry. Available online at http://www.bristol-inquiry.org.uk/

vii Weick K, Sutcliffe K, Quinn R, *Managing the Unexpected: Assuring High Performance in an Age of Complexity.* San Francisco. Jossey-Bass, 2001.

generally assume that problems will occur and they have the systems in place to cope with these problems early on.[vi]

Importance of co-evolving with ongoing changes

In order to survive, health care systems need to continually change and evolve. They need to match the demands of individual patients, of their communities' needs and values and with the most recent technological advances.

This co-evolution also needs to take into account the change in the health care teams themselves. As individuals and relationships alter within teams so will the way in which they provide health care. For instance, a nurse and doctor who get on well will in all likelihood give a different type of care from another team where their relationship is poor.

Health care systems work at many levels; both within the context of a larger system like the NHS and then as trusts, local hospitals or the village primary care team. Change is going to happen at all these levels and there will be important effects of changes between these systems. The different systems need to co-evolve with each other. Whilst a village has its own defined network, it also has a relationship with the broader political context and thence back to the Department of Health and the NHS as a whole. Change cannot therefore be determined in isolation. In order to maintain the values or culture of the local hospital, the larger Trust and NHS will have to allow it to adapt and evolve to meet local needs, some of which do not necessarily meet national plans.

Capability for change

How will health care systems be able to cope with this complicated mess? Generally through focusing on the development of personal and organisational capability rather than detailed competency. This issue was highlighted in the recommendations of the Bristol Inquiry. Although the recommendations describe broadening competency, it is clear from the description that what was recommended is the need to build the capability of the NHS workforce, including the need for capable team working and clear leadership.[vii] One challenge is to manage the tension between reducing the rigidities (to allow innovation) while maintaining high standards and quality of care.

Agile systems can be defined as being capable of doing new and unfamiliar tasks in unfamiliar and changing environments. They are capable of delivering different types of care to different types of patients. Their constant adaptability and ability to evolve with their environment means they will always survive; albeit in different forms. In essence they are constantly learning from what goes on about them.

Principles for thriving in unpredictable times

1. **Deliver purpose, focus and commitment**; in complex adaptive systems, the inefficiencies that are perceived often result from different players in the system holding different sets of motivations, purpose and focus for the work. Ensuring there is a clear vision of how the patient should experience care can minimise movement away from the original solution and may even help ensure continuous improvement.

2. **Be sensitive to the environment through feedback**; provide all those involved with the improved process plenty of information about performance and issues. Empowered adaptive agents, armed with the right information, can ensure swift and flexible responses to problems. The valves in the oil refinery pipeline need to wait for instruction; with purposeful feedback health care practitioners can get on with making improvements with no central direction.

3. **Be ready for change**; as we have described, change is inevitable. The key to a sustainable organisation is one that is ready for change and that understands the unpredictable nature of what might happen. Freezing the improved process with strict procedures and other limitations will not guarantee sustainability or stop individuals going back to the 'old' way. Complex adaptive systems constantly change and develop, co-evolving with other changes going on at the time. Redesigned processes need to be allowed to continue to evolve and develop free of hindrances.

4. **Ensure slack**; Change needs capacity, a system that is constantly working to full capacity has no ability to change or evolve. Natural models show that in order to evolve with the environment, slack is needed to allow for some wastage.

viii Zimmerman B, Lindberg C, Plsek P, *Edgeware; Insights from Complexity Science for Health care Leaders*, Texas: VHA Inc, 1998.

5. **Emphasise team working;** adaptive systems are as effective as the relationships and interactions between the members of the system. Paying attention to these connections, growing them, supporting them and sustaining them, can help maintain and develop improvements.

6. **Encourage capability;** develop individuals within teams to be capable of working in unfamiliar environments and with unfamiliar tasks.

7. **Listen to the 'expert';** the people who know most about what is happening and what is changing are the people actually doing it. Therefore, the most successful organisations at surviving are those that have mechanisms for learning from the front line and constantly adapting and changing to what is needed.

8. **Work across boundaries;** care is care and for many patients it doesn't matter who provides what and which budget it comes from. An agile system works across boundaries, blurring the margins of who does what, doing what is needed at the time (the doctor takes blood to save the patient another journey, the district nurse collects the wife's medication whilst getting the new dressing for the husband; sharing the results of assessments done by different professions and agencies, health visitors treating illnesses as well as giving advice). Encourage teams to think outside their work environment to network with other care givers (the housing agency, the school), ensuring the best care system is offered to the patient (would contraceptive advice come best from a teacher?).

9. **Don't simplify;** 'things' happen in health care for many complicated reasons. This applies equally to success as to failure. Simplifying the analysis of why things happen ignores the true complexity of systems. By accepting the complicated nature of events and what leads up to them, innovative thinking and deeper understanding in preparation for future events is encouraged.

10. **Listen to the shadow system;**[viii] informal relationships, gossip and rumour hold the key to understanding how others perceive the issues and task in hand. Management objectives and processes that ignore these are unlikely to be successful.

Conclusion

Health care systems need to constantly co-evolve. This co-evolution occurs at many levels within the health care system and alongside many other systems (the individual patient, the community etc.). Survival is only possible through this constant process of co-evolution. In order to survive and be able to evolve, health care systems need to build capability to work in unfamiliar environments, doing unfamiliar tasks. This can only occur through the development of the people and teams within the health care system and the infrastructure needed to help them do their job well. A key issue is the building of capability within the health service rather than designing mechanistic but competent systems that are unable to adapt.

3 | Planning and scheduling: maintaining flow in adaptive systems

David J. Yarrow, Sarah W. Fraser, Barry Tennison

Why scheduling health care activities is so difficult

As the authors of the previous chapter have illustrated, health care is difficult to predict, if not impossible, and complex in nature. This chapter seeks to help you consider the management of the 'flow' of patients as a means of achieving agile practice.

Non-linearity and lack of predictability are the main reasons why scheduling is so difficult in health care. Add to this the wide variety of types of care, the different professions, organisations and teams that all have their own operating standards and the challenge becomes obvious. The impact is more people waiting longer for care that is variable in terms of both process and outcome.

While it has its own unique characteristics, health care is not alone in facing difficulties in scheduling its activities. For example, much of manufacturing industry, whilst often thought of as being like a production line, is actually closer to the 'jobbing shop' – a term used to describe a production facility which is willing and able to make a wide variety of different things. For some manufacturers, far from a series of identical products flowing down a production line, each 'job' is unique – they may all be made from the same material, for example, and have the same basic form, but each new customer wants a different shape and size, different characteristics, perhaps a quantity of only one, or at the most several.

The extreme case is the wrought-iron worker, who will make you a gate for your front drive, a banister for your staircase, a pair of decorative candlesticks for your lounge. He'll make them to order, to your specification. As volumes grow, he'll employ others to help him. Now they start competing for the equipment and materials in the workshop, and decisions have to be made in real time about which customer's order should take priority, which needs the experienced expert and which can be delegated to the junior employee, and so on.

In health care, the general practitioner experiences a similar (or perhaps even greater) level of variety and complexity of task. In one afternoon he might deal with a patient who is having difficulty stabilising their warfarin dose, a tired child with an anxious mother, conflicting medications, phoning test results to patients, comforting a bereaved relative, and so on.

In this chapter, we will draw parallels between some health care systems and some work systems in other settings, in an attempt to shed new light on both the challenges we face in health care and some techniques which have been found useful elsewhere which just might have something to offer.

Are we being served?

A common, and understandable, reaction to discussions about manufacturing-based approaches is 'Yes, but health care systems aren't like factories.' We'll return to this thought later, but in the meantime let's also recognise that there are also parallels with many service-oriented systems. A restaurant, for example, copes with a similar level of unpredictability to that experienced in some health care settings. Who knows how many customers will walk through the door in the next hour? Or what they will order? We may try to bring order and predictability by operating a reservations system, even by asking diners to pre-order their food, but how do we cope when a party turns up late, or brings two extra diners without warning, or when someone changes their mind about what they want to eat, or when the kitchen equipment fails just after they arrive?

At some levels, this sounds rather like a primary care practice that has to deal with patients who don't turn up for appointments, last minute requests for urgent appointments, and patients who prefer to see the doctor for their immunisation, rather than the nurse running the travel clinic.

Professional practices also provide some interesting and potentially useful parallels with health care. The experienced lawyer is a highly valued resource, in great demand from her practice's systems and staff. She is often pulled in several directions at once, and asked to be in many different places with too little time in between. What if a court case is delayed, or takes longer than expected, and the lawyer is due back at the office to meet another important client? Which client should take priority? Who could cover for the absent lawyer? And who can make these decisions, trying to find the optimum trade-offs in a highly complex and ever-changing situation?

This scenario is replicated in health care systems as different professional groups interact with each other and patients in ways that are complex and non-linear. Add to this the contested models of care, differing perceptions between patients and staff and conflicting requirements in terms of cost and outcome, and decision-making in health care really does look like a thorny business and not one that lends itself to easily recognisable improvements.

For example, in response to the frustration of cancellation of elective treatments when emergency pressures rise, some hospitals have tried to separate out capacity for the two types of care. The results of this have been mixed and many have found they have experienced a greater pressure on the reduced emergency capacity, especially at unexpected times, and less than optimum usage of elective capacity.

Despite scheduling appointments being such a difficult task and even though there are some long waiting times for certain types of care, it is interesting to note that the majority of the several million activities underway in the NHS every day, are scheduled effectively, albeit sometimes inefficiently. They do take place in ways that allow patients to progress along pathways of care, whether explicit or not. This is part of the inherent order (self-organisation) of the health care system.

The challenge for agile health care systems is to take the difficulties and discover ways to plan and schedule care so that it is efficient, meets the patient's needs, is cost effective and yet maintains the ability to flex and adapt to the ever-changing pressures on a day-to-day basis. Health care is not alone in facing this challenge, nor is it alone in having failed so far to overcome it comprehensively. However, in some health care settings, and in some other sectors, advances have been made, and they are worth examining to see whether they have something useful to offer.

Differentiating planning from scheduling

It is important to distinguish between 'planning' and 'scheduling'. We can plan to equip a restaurant with kitchens, furniture and staff capable of serving 100 customers in an evening. We can plan its opening hours, buy food and arrange staff hours on the assumption that the diners and their demands will follow certain patterns. We can even build in contingencies to allow for the fact that we know there is some uncertainty about the accuracy of those assumptions. The plans may be carefully constructed, the assumptions based on research, analysis of history, predictions of customers' behaviours.

Scheduling, however, is something rather different from planning. Scheduling is an activity that comes into its own when the action begins. The first 20 customers have arrived. They arrived in quite a rush, and now they're all placing orders with their waiters. What will they choose from the menu? What if their choices make competing demands on the kitchen staff and equipment? Table 1 wants three soups and 2 melon boats. The soups are ready, but the melon boats need some preparation. The sous-chef starts the job, but then another order arrives from table 10. They only want one melon boat, so if they took the first one we could serve them now. But that would mean table 1 waiting a bit longer. And so on. The scheduling activity is never-ending, until closing time comes around.

If the planning we did in advance was effective, then the scheduling will be easier. If we could provide a perfectly accurate forecast in advance, predicting exact timings and choices for every diner, then the schedule would be cast in stone before the first diners arrived, and the kitchen would run like clockwork. However, real life isn't like that.

In health care systems this becomes even more complex. Usually planning is an annual activity focused on maintaining services and activity levels and there may be some requirements to improve efficiency built into this process. Access to services is impacted by plans for workforce development, equipment purchase, changes in clinical practice and so on.

In comparison, the scheduling is more immediate, with the month-to-month, day-to-day managing the process of health care activities left to practitioners and administrators. The complexities of interaction and tensions between managerial and clinical decision-making ensure this is a task that is difficult to achieve in an effective and efficient way.

Planning is often associated with the setting of targets. Whilst performance goals are useful, they can have undesirable effects on the system if they are not matched with effort to improve the scheduling arrangements. For example, in the NHS, imposing maximum waiting times with managerial pressure on individuals has led to falsification of records, invention of categories of 'non-waiting', and some patients receiving poorer treatment.[i] Targets and pressures inevitably influence the behaviours of those who are in the thick of the action. If you tell me that a patient must not remain at a certain point in the process more than an hour, I'm likely to find a way to make sure they move after 55 minutes – even if the act of making this happen is wasting time I could be spending doing something more useful, and is of no help whatsoever to the patient.

[i] National Audit Office. *Inappropriate adjustments to NHS waiting lists.* London: The Stationery Office, 2001.

Coping with detail

If you've ever visited a weather station – one of those remote little huts, covered in instruments, where they monitor weather patterns and provide the data that feed the weather forecasts – you may have been told that 'We never actually get the weather wrong, just the timing. The rain we predicted for yesterday afternoon did come along, it just took a bit longer than we thought, so it fell while you were asleep and you didn't see it.'

This may be true, but it's not very helpful. It does, however, illustrate a point.

In the real world, the only thing that we know for certain about a forecast is that it's very unlikely to be precisely right. And the greater the detail, the more scope there is for variation. For example, you can predict how many balls they'll draw in the National Lottery next Saturday, and you'll be right. You can predict with a high degree of confidence that at least one of the numbers will have a '7' in it. If you could predict what all of the numbers would be, that would be quite something, but the chance of that is about the same as the chance of stopping a complete stranger in the street and correctly guessing their telephone number, code and all.

This is why we need to schedule, as well as plan. History, statistics and analysis can give us a fairly reliable prediction of the 'high level' patterns of demand and activity, but, as they say, the devil is in the detail.

There is a strong temptation, faced with the task of managing a complicated system, to try to control it in more and more detailed ways (especially when it does not respond as wished). This is analogous to *reductionism* in philosophy: the belief that a system can be understood by understanding its parts, and that if its behaviour is not understood, we need to study the parts in even greater detail. Various threads in philosophy run counter to this, and imply that understanding may be impossible, or achieved

ii Taylor FW, 'Shop management' in *Scientific Management*, Harper & Row: USA, 1964 (original article written in 1911).

only by standing back (or above). For adaptive systems, this suggests looking for the emergent phenomena, properties and patterns, and the overall responses to pressure, rather than trying to increase the detail about the elements and their interactions.

Looking to manufacturing industry for some lessons, there are plenty to be found, although many of them seem to be about what not to do. In the history of manufacturing, the names F.W. Taylor and Henry Ford loom large.[ii] Taylor's contribution is known as 'Scientific Management', which grew from the belief that perfection in production systems would be achieved by breaking down the overall task into smaller and smaller elements, studying each element in minute detail and re-designing the task for efficiency and repeatability, as well as training and assigning workers as specialists in very specific tasks. Work measurement techniques were developed which could define the time that a task would take (or should take) in incredible detail, right down to every movement of a limb and every press of a button. Standards were set and people's performance was measured against them, with incentives for those who could meet (or even beat) the standard times. The theory was wonderful. The system would be perfected, the productivity maximised, planning and scheduling would become a science rather than an art!

The past tense is actually misleading. This approach is still applied in many industries, and it would be wrong to say that it has been wholly unsuccessful. In the main, however, it seems that attempts to reduce and control are ultimately doomed to fail. People are people, not machines. Things happen – materials arrive late, equipment breaks down, people do things differently, incentives have unforeseen effects, demand patterns don't match the forecast, and so on. Above all, we have come to realise that variation is an inherent feature of any process, perhaps especially when human beings are an inherent part of that process. If you don't believe this, try measuring the time it takes you to get to work each morning, and see if it is always the same. Or try throwing a dart at a dartboard. If you're a good player, sometimes you can hit the bull's-eye. But can you do it every time, no matter how hard you try to do everything exactly the same as the last time?

In scheduling terms, the end result is that, even if we could predict demand precisely (which we never can), if we base our schedules on our estimates and predictions of how long each activity in a process will take to complete, before long we will find that the combination of large numbers of small variations will produce some effects which are very different from what we expected. Table 1 shows how small differences compound with

Table 1: Probability of a reliable process for each process step

No. of steps in the process	Initial probability 0.95	Initial probability 0.99
1	0.950	0.99
25	0.280	0.98
50	0.080	0.95
100	0.006	0.90

each step in the process. Even with a high initial probability of a reliable and controlled process (95%), after just 25 steps, the probability of a successful outcome (such as a precise prediction of the time taken) is significantly diminished (28%).

One of the challenges for health care processes is reliability. In a complex adaptive system it is likely there will be frequent changes happening to the individuals in the system. For example, a new consultant may join the team, the expert booking clerk may leave, a patient's need to be seen may become more urgent, a vital piece of equipment may break and there may be no funds to replace it quickly. These are everyday occurrences and the scheduling system will need to adapt in some way to solve the problems. Reliability concerns more than the smooth functioning and flow of the process. It also involves making tacit behaviours more explicit.

For example, a particular elective unit ran well largely because a particular nursing sister took to herself the task of screening patients, two weeks before their admission, for factors (like co-existing illness) which could lead to their treatment not being possible on the day. She would then take action so that the patient would be treated and/or rescheduled. This role 'emerged' because of the favourable environment in the unit, towards initiative and professional respect. What would happen if the sister moved off the unit, and was replaced by someone else? Would the crucial but informal screening process be replicated?

The limited value of 'work-in-progress'

All of these issues and challenges manifest themselves in manufacturing environments, and have been the focus of a great deal of effort by a lot of people for a very long time. If manufacturing managers have focused sooner on these problems, or with greater resources, this is at least partly because when a scheduling system

iii Cheng TCE, Podolsky S, *Just-in-Time Manufacturing – an Introduction*, Chapman & Hall, London, 1993.

in a factory doesn't perform well, the results are extremely visible. Before long, the nice clean, ordered factory is awash with bits of material and half-finished products that seem to have nowhere to go. They were scheduled to move on to the next stage in the process, but the schedule turns out to have been wrong. So they begin to pile up all over the place.

In the manufacturing parlance, this is described as a build-up of 'work-in-progress' (often abbreviated to 'wip'). Actually, human nature being what it is, there is a tendency for individuals working away deep in the heart of the factory to be comforted by seeing a pile of 'wip' all around them. This means that they know they'll be able to keep working, even if (as often happens) there is an interruption to the supply of parts or products from previous stages in the process. This can be important to the majority of people, whose desire is to do a good job and who really don't want to be standing idle waiting for problems elsewhere to be solved. In some cases, financial rewards depend on being able to keep busy, providing an additional reason to be comforted by some 'just in case' work in progress.

A build up of 'work in progress' is also a feature of many health care systems, demonstrated by the lists of people waiting for an appointment or treatment, as well as the piles of patients' notes in the consultant's office, waiting for the letters to be typed, appointments arranged etc. Such build-ups are often seen as an inevitable side-effect of the demands on the system. But is this really always the case? Is a queue, or some other accumulation of people or paperwork, ever created deliberately in the belief that this is a good way of making the system work, and guarding against uncertainty?

In the last twenty years the message has spread through manufacturing industry that such 'just in case' approaches are counter-productive, and must be replaced by 'just in time'.iii The key principle here is that the flow of work should occur through 'pull' rather than 'push' mechanisms. Surrounding ourselves with queues of work waiting to be done is a way of hiding our problems, certainly not a way of solving them.

An experienced production manager, who has spent much of her recent working life 'draining' the system of excessive wip in order to reveal and then tackle root causes of problems, might feel a sense of déjà vu when she turns up for an out-patients appointment to find she is one of 10 people who have all been given the same appointment time and must now sit and wait … and wait … for no apparent reason. In some production systems, the application of such 'push' principles has meant that material is typically only having value added to it for 5 to 10% of the time it spends in the factory. The other 90% is spent being moved, checked, reorganised and, mostly, just sitting around waiting for something to happen. In advanced production systems that have tackled this issue, value-adding time can be 50% or even much higher than that.

In the health care setting, 'non-value-added time' becomes an issue for human beings, rather than materials, and has implications both for outcomes and for the quality of the user's experience. So a low ratio (in terms of time spent in useful 'value-adding' parts of the health care process versus time spent on non-useful activity) might be even more problematic than in the factory setting. Well, a recent study[iv] of two Accident and Emergency departments investigated precisely this ratio. Guess what – it found that, typically, 'value-adding time' was less than 25% of the total patient throughput time.

So, planning and scheduling in health care systems is a complex, messy and unpredictable business, mirroring the experience in many production environments. In what way can the concepts of agility support the design of processes that meet the needs of patients, practitioners, managers and funders?

Levels of health care scheduling systems

All hospitals and primary care practices operate basic scheduling systems as standard. Some have participated in quality and process improvement projects to redesign their processes and speed up the flow of patients, reduce waste and remove non-value added activities. If these projects have been successful, these systems can be said to have reached the *lean* level.

The next stage for organisations is to aspire to be *agile*. This means they cannot rely on rigid procedures and protocols to keep the process working reliably. Instead they need to ensure sufficient feedback and monitoring, common goals and personal engagement of staff and patients in the scheduling issues, so that they can continue to deliver customised services, efficiently. See Table 2 overleaf.

Understanding predictability

One of the key issues for scheduling is when there is little agreement or certainty amongst the stakeholders on the nature of the

iv Modernisation Agency, *Ideal Design of Emergency Access (IDEA) Programme: National Report*, Modernisation Agency, 2002 (January)

[v] Murray M 'Patient Care: Access', *BMJ*, 320:1594–1596, 2000.

[vi] Stacey R, *Strategic Management and Organisational Dynamics; the challenge of complexity*, 3rd Edition London: Financial Times, 1999.

Table 2: Levels of health care scheduling systems

1: Basic	• Scheduling system is in place • Some policies and procedures concerned with scheduling • Operational conflict between urgent and more routine activities that impact negatively on the schedules • Although some improvement has been made, there are still delays in access and in carrying out routine activities such as elective operations • Reliance on one-off activities to correct scheduling imbalances (long waiters)
2: Lean	• Efforts in place to manage demand • Capacity planning in place • Most delay anticipated in advance and efforts made to correct poor scheduling • Unpredictable issues and events need to be discussed with a wide variety of stakeholders • Eliminated the year end push to reduce waiting lists • Waste elimination has produced at least 15% more capacity • Pulling demand though the acute care system
3: Agile	• Quick change-overs (theatre utilisation) • Doing today's work today[v] • Rescheduling done cooperatively with stakeholders, patients and carers, to suit their needs • Flexibility to provide special teams at short notice • Synchronised scheduling throughout the local health care system; principles of 'pull' rather than 'push' are applied to good effect • Care is coordinated to meet the needs of the specific patient, not as part of a mass customisation of pathways

problem or its solution and where the results are not predictable in detail. For example, in creating a way for older people to enjoy coherent and coordinated services provided by both health and social care departments, a linear approach is unlikely to be a successful tactic, at least at the outset.

The relationship between certainty, agreement and complexity is given in Figure 2.[vi] In general:

• when operating in the *simple* zone, relatively straightforward and common management techniques can be effective, if done well: for example, project management, process re-engineering or constraint analysis

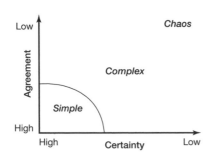

Figure 2

- when operating in the zone of *chaos,* one cannot expect too much from purely managerial efforts: it may be best to scan for patterns and changes (especially in the external environment) and search out alternative ways of looking at the system, in some cases even acting fairly randomly on it to disturb the pattern of attractors[vii]

- the zone of *complexity* is the challenge for those leading health care and indeed in other parts of the public and private sectors: here it may be best to build connections and networks; enhance communication; work collectively on minimum specifications; listen to the shadow system, working with paradox; and be prepared to take multiple actions, allowing direction to emerge.

Where agreement and certainty are high, processes are usually more predictable; here planning and control is an effective management activity.[viii] It is here that basic scheduling is crucial. For example, most stakeholders in the process agree on the most useful process to diagnose lung cancer and have a high level of certainty that the process achieves its objective.

However, many NHS service delivery processes start out with little agreement or certainty about the problem or solution. Here it is important for leaders and project managers alike to recognise that they are not able to, and should not be expected to, figure out the solution. Rather, they should spend time in discussion, creating connections, team building, enabling dialogue, and creating the space for the system's natural creativity to work. An important activity is the generation and agreement of goals and direction of travel. Managers and leaders are part of the system, not objective observers, so their behaviour is also important and will have an impact, favourably or otherwise, on outcomes.

After years of 'efficiency savings', much of the NHS is already 'lean' and can boast that it wastes very little. Unfortunately, this efficiency has been bought at the cost of leaving little room for experimentation and learning. But to handle unpredictable times, a major requirement is the ability to try new directions and techniques, and the space to learn from them. This is, for example, one basis of the idea of improvement collaboratives and the plan-do-study-act (PDSA) cycle.[ix] There is a need to engender a mindset that takes advantage of any 'troughs' in the schedule to practise the disciplines of PDSA, and implants the capability to do so. There is a need to recognise that systems can not run day after day, month after month, year after year at the limits of their

[vii] Wheatley M, *Leadership and the New Science.* Berrett-Koehler Publishers Inc 2001.

[viii] Plsek PE, Greenhalgh P, The challenge of complexity in health care, *BMJ,* 323:625–8, 2001.

[ix] Fraser SW, Burch K, Knightley M, Osborne M, Wilson A, 'Using collaborative improvement in a single organisation: improving anticoagulant care', *International Journal for Health Care Quality Assurance,* 15(4, 5), 2002.

capacity, and be expected to continue to function effectively, much less to be capable of adaptation and improvement. Indeed, a system that possesses a small amount of 'surplus' capacity, in which the space thus created is used to good effect to focus on improvement activity, will in the long run become far more effective and efficient than a system which is continually 'running on empty'.

What has worked elsewhere?

Let's return to the thought that some ideas developed in manufacturing industry may be helpful as health care re-examines its approaches to planning and scheduling, in a bid to become leaner, more agile, more effective, and to improve and maintain *flow*. What characterises manufacturing settings in which such progress has been made?

A common theme is that, in these settings, those who seek to *improve* the work processes have first focused their efforts on *understanding* them. What is really going on in our process as it exists today? What leads us to plan and schedule activities and events in the way that we do – upon what beliefs are we basing the plans, and what is our theory or model of how our plans will translate into reality? And, crucially, what actually happens in practice? If the plan was that a certain number of products would be completed (or diners served, or patients treated) in a certain time period, how did this compare with the reality of what actually occurred? And, likewise, if our schedule suggested that product A would be ready for dispatch to the customer at time t_A (and product B at time t_B, and product C at time t_C) was this actually what happened?

Some key themes in such a quest for understanding are *triggers*, and *signals*, and *flows*, and *constraints*. When we act to set another product off on its journey through the factory (or a patient on their journey through our system), what is the trigger that leads us to do so at a particular point in time? And what signals do we send to others that lead them to play their parts in particular ways? And what are the characteristics of the way materials and products (or customers, or patients) *flow* through our processes? What enables that flow to be smooth and fast, and conversely what can interrupt it, causing it to be unpredictable, uneven, and perhaps slower than we wished or predicted? Crucially, what are the *constraints* which determine the realities of when a product arrives at the factory's exit door (or 'finished goods bay', as they are often known), as opposed to the time that our schedule said that this *should*

Box 3: *Push* versus *pull*

A characteristic of many well-established and well-intentioned scheduling approaches is that, once the schedule has been worked out, those who are managing the process will do everything in their power to adhere to it. The schedule says that the next product should be moved from location 1 to location 2 at 3:00pm, so that's what we will do. The fact that location 2 houses a machine that has broken down, and now has a queue of unprocessed material in front of it, is probably invisible to us, and in any case would be irrelevant. The schedule is king! If the schedule says move, you move! The schedule is *pushing*, and the more it pushes, the faster we'll make some progress.

Er ... not quite, actually. It is now well-established that, where circumstances allow, an approach which *pulls* material through a production system has many advantages over its *push*-based equivalent. This is often counter-intuitive for people brought up with an obsession for high equipment utilisation, thorough planning and strict adherence to the schedule. But the fact is that progress is quicker, quality better, efficiency higher and adaptability and improvability much enhanced in pull-based systems.[x,xi,xii,xiii]

[x] Schonberger RJ, *World Class Manufacturing – the Lessons of Simplicity Applied*, The Free Press, New York, 1986.

[xi] Monden Y, *Toyota Production System – Practical Approach to Production Management*, Industrial Engineering and Management Press, Norcorss, Georgia, 1983.

[xii] Hanson P, Voss CA, Blackmon K, Oak B, *Made in Europe, A Four Nations Best Practice Study*, IBM UK Ltd/London Business School, Warwick/London, 1994.

[xiii] Womack JP, Jones DT, *Lean Thinking*, Touchstone Books, London, 1996.

happen? Indeed, are there any such constraints? (The answer to this last question, by the way, is YES! There are constraints in any system, at any time, and recognising them and dealing with them is one of the keys to understanding and improving the system.)

Once a broad understanding of the system or process is achieved, various specific techniques may be seen to be applicable. In manufacturing settings, a common theme has been the application of techniques that switch the scheduling emphasis from *push* to *pull*. How this is done depends on the physical and logistical characteristics of the process in question, but a common and very effective technique is the use of signals from one resource (e.g. a machine or a person) to indicate either 'I'm busy at the moment, don't send me any more work to do until I tell you I'm ready for it' or, conversely, 'I've finished all the work that's available to me ... please send me something else to do!' This sounds so simple that it's almost facile – but *that's the point!* The best ideas are the simple ones, and for all that this one is really simple in principle, in practice it's not always so simple to implement. Pull principles can be enacted through signalling devices that are sometimes called 'kanbans' (consisting of lights that are on for 'stop' or off for 'go'; or the arrival of a 'kanban card' that signifies 'send me the next one', while its absence signifies 'Do nothing till you hear from me!'; or other similar devices). The reason they're called 'kanbans' is that the idea originated in Japan, and 'kanban' is Japanese for (wait for it!) 'signal'. It is such a simple idea, but can be incredibly effective in transforming processes that have become difficult to manage and are under-performing, into ones that perform at unprecedented levels and display their further potential for improvement for all to see.

Another common and powerful theme is the discovery of a process's *constraints*, and refinement of the scheduling system to deal with them. There's an old saying that 'every chain has a weakest link', and the same is true of systems and processes – they always contain constraints. A constraint is a resource that cannot do its job as quickly as the other resources in the process. Think of it as the neck of a bottle – the liquid can only flow out of the bottle at the speed that it can flow through the narrowest part of the bottle, the neck. In a factory setting, the constraint may well be a machine. If the production machinery can fill cans of soup at a rate of 1000 per hour, but the labelling machine can only stick on labels at a rate of 500 per hour, what is the maximum number of finished (and labelled) cans of soup that can emerge from the factory in an hour? The answer is obvious – 500. However, in more complex production systems, it's often nothing like that obvious. In fact, very often, the constraint (or constraints) are completely invisible and change identity from time to time depending on things like the particular 'mix' of products being made. This might explain why, in the absence of an understanding of what constrains our rate of production, we resort to pushing as much raw material as possible into the front end of the factory, in the vain hope that the more we push, the faster finished products will emerge at the other end!

Such an approach can have some unfortunate consequences, which are fairly predictable when you stop and think abut them. Remember those Tom and Jerry cartoons, when someone is standing on a hose-pipe while someone else turns the tap on harder and harder, pumping more and more water into one end of the hose-pipe while only a dribble is emerging at the other end. What happens to the hose-pipe immediately 'upstream' from the constraint? It bulges, of course! The pressure builds and builds, until eventually something has to give, and the pipe bursts. Walk around a few factories with an educated eye, looking for critical constraint resources, and you may find you can spot them quite easily. They're the ones where the queue of material waiting to be processed has become so big that it might be touching the ceiling, or spilling over into the walkways that are supposed to be kept clear for people! Yet what does our scheduling system do? It keeps right on pushing! And the machines that receive the material first (which are 'upstream' of the constraint) keep gobbling up the work enthusiastically, so the scheduling system just pushes the constraint all the more!

Every chain has a weakest link, and guess where the chain breaks when it gets stretched far enough.

Health care systems are no different – they all contain their constraints too. And just like in many production systems, the people managing the processes are often blissfully unaware of the disproportionate influence that these critical resources are having on the entire system. They may be pieces of equipment (an X-ray machine) or they may be people (a triage nurse). They may be obvious and well known to all concerned, or they may be invisible and apparently (deceptively) unimportant. What is for sure is that they are there, and if we are not focusing on them as we plan and schedule our activities, then they are likely to be almost solely responsible for the fact that all those lovely plans and schedules, just like our dreams, never quite come true!

Just like the idea of 'pull not push', the thinking expounded above is really rather simple but has tended to be totally absent from most well-established approaches to planning and scheduling. It was first revealed to the manufacturing community by a man called Eli Goldratt in his seminal book[xiv] *The Goal* in the 1980s, and is now commonly referred to as the 'Theory of Constraints'.[xv] Notoriously harder to apply than it is to understand, TOC is a powerful bit of thoughtware that has influenced many (though by no means all) production scheduling systems for the better, and is beginning to do the same for many in other sectors, including health care.

The principles of *pull scheduling* and application of the *Theory of Constraints* are just two sets of ideas that have made a major impact outside of health care and could perhaps have much to offer as those who manage health care systems and processes seek new ways to improve them. Neither is a panacea, nor could be easily applied or necessarily applicable in every case. However, experience in manufacturing systems suggests that these ideas are well worth exploring, and could make a big difference if intelligently applied.

[xiv] Goldratt EM, Cox J, *The Goal*, Gower, Aldershot, 1984.

[xv] Goldratt EM, *What is this Thing Called Theory of Constraints and How Should it be Implemented?* Croton-on-Hudson, N.Y.: North River Press, 1990.

4 | Reducing work in progress and waste

David J. Yarrow, Steve Unwin

A patient's journey in Utopia?

Picture the scene. A patient arrives one morning at the clinic. She is immediately welcomed into a consulting room by a professional (A) who has ample time to listen, discuss and explain, and to arrive at a provisional diagnosis that requires the patient to undergo a series of tests. These can be arranged immediately, and the patient finds herself minutes later in another room with another professional (B), who puts her at her ease and proceeds to administer the tests. Some laboratory analysis is required, which will take about an hour, so the patient has time to get a snack before returning for the feedback. B is available to talk her through the results and their implications. Treatment is required. It can be started today. It is convenient for the patient to stay a little longer, so arrangements are made and before she knows it she is with professional C, discussing her treatment and, shortly afterwards, beginning it. An hour later, she is on her way home, feeling well-informed about the diagnosis and prognosis, and satisfied that the treatment is underway. She has an appointment to return in 3 weeks, at a time she has chosen, to see C again for a follow-up consultation.

Is this realistic? We're sure it happens, but we're not sure that it's typical. This is the real world we're living in. This unit didn't just have one patient to deal with today, it had fifty. And A, B and C weren't just sitting around waiting for this patient to turn up, so they could spring into action and help her along on her smooth, uninterrupted, idealised patient journey. In the real world there are queues, imbalances, backlogs and delays. We'd all love to treat every patient as a unique individual, and provide them all with the perfect 'service' they crave, but let's get real!

Those 'interested' patients and visitors with grease in the soles of their shoes

Do you recognise the type? They're 'interested' in what's going on around them as they wait for their X-ray, or as the patient they're accompanying is explaining that she has to go home without having her operation because something went wrong or someone else has had to take priority. They might engage you in conversation about *schedules* and *queues* and *lead times* and *expediting*. Their vocabulary seems odd but they appear to have some idea what they're talking about. Another clue to their identity is that they're probably quite interested in the equipment too, figuring out what it does and why it bleeps like that every now and then.

These are the Production People. They have jobs in companies that make things, and to them a hospital seems kind of like a factory, similar but different in a funny sort of a way; a fascinating sort of a way.

Their reactions to what they see in the hospital could go either way. Most of them work in production facilities that suffer their fair share of disruption and overload, where carefully-designed plans rarely resemble reality very closely, and the daily routine includes a fair degree of uncertainty, re-scheduling and fire-fighting to overcome the delays, the shortages and the unexpected events. The chances are that they'll be generally sympathetic to the problems you're up against, and explain to Aunty (the patient) that in a big, complex organisation like this 'stuff happens' – it's not as easy as you'd imagine to get it running like clockwork.

On the other hand, a few of them might see things a bit differently. They work in one of those rather superior factories, where things run a bit more smoothly and there's an air of efficiency and predictability. They might suggest to you that there must be a better way than this. Some of them will mutter strange stuff about 'lean production', 'kanban' and 'reducing the wip', but they probably won't be inclined to explain themselves.

Time to come out of the closet. You've guessed by now anyway. We're two of those strange Production People. We've got certificates to prove it, though it's a while since we spent much time on a shop floor. Anyway, in this chapter we're going to try to translate some of our Production People gobbledegook into English, and hope that this might help us all to work out whether we can really learn anything from it that could help health care systems to be more agile.

A parallel universe?

We Production People dream of Utopia too. The theory is simple – a customer wants one of our products, so let's make one for him and gratefully take his money. Trouble is, he wants it tomorrow. Now, in theory, it would only take 5 hours to make it – 2 hours of work on machine X, 1 hour on machine Y, an hour being painted by person Z, an hour to dry then it's ready. But the machines are all busy already, even if we could get the paperwork raised straight away. In fact they've all got queues in front of them. We could do a bit of progress chasing, which would help, but machine X is busy with one of our type 2 products (what we want is a type 1), so there'll be an extra half hour while the set-up is changed, and then we'll get stick from our colleagues who are trying to chase the type 2s through because customers are waiting for them too. Then the whole thing might have to be repeated at machine Y. And, of course, the paint-spray equipment is doing red today, but we want blue. They usually set it up for blue on Thursdays, and persuading them to switch to blue for a one-off is impossible (we've tried that one before! You can't blame them really; it's an hour-long job to clean one colour out of the spray equipment and start with another colour). All in all there is no way we can achieve what the customer is asking. That 'theoretical' 5 hours looks more like 5 days in practice.

Manufacturing industry: 100 years of learning

The process of change is an ongoing one, a journey. Many of the changes have become embedded as second nature within production organisations, but many served their purpose for a time and then were superseded as new pressures, new thinking and new ideas took their place. The journey is a story of steps taken. Some of them were short-lived and perhaps served to overcome a particular obstacle or meet the special needs of a given time or environment. Other steps have delivered changes that have been maintained for longer periods of time. Even these long-lived steps should not be thought of as permanent since this change process and the journey continues. In a book written in ten years time, we must expect that the leading-edge techniques described in this book have either become embedded or replaced if we are not to be believe that continuous improvement has faltered.

Like the health care process, the manufacturing process is one of bringing the right people, equipment, methods and materials together in the right place at the right time. Equally, it is important to do it cost effectively and efficiently to produce a product at a price that will sell and produce a profit.

In the early part of the last century many of the basic characteristics of production environments had been established. Mass production methods had seen a shift of manufacturing away from reliance on craftsmanship to create individual products, to mass production of large numbers of identical and interchangeable products. The manufacture of motor cars is a good example of this change. The world was hungry for these products and even into the 1950s and 1960s manufacturers found ready markets for their products almost irrespective of their quality. Customers were prepared to join waiting lists to purchase products that they expected would be unreliable and subject to defects. The thrill of simply obtaining these products after a period of austerity was joy enough for most customers. Manufacturers were under little pressure to develop and improve products and were consequently lethargic at introducing change. From the late 1960s onwards things began to change. Japanese products, once the byword for poor quality, began to appear with unrivalled levels of reliability and performance. Customers started to become more discerning. From being glad to receive any kind of product, they now demanded both better quality and better value. The pressure to improve began to be felt. Though some areas and industries would initially resist, this pressure became inexorable and has spread over time into many areas that thirty years ago were completely isolated from such pressures.

In health care, as in production, the challenge created by this customer demand resembles a balancing act with each decision having positive and negative impacts. In the production environment, make more items in a batch and unit costs come down as you save on setting-up costs. However you have the costs of more material in use and a longer wait before switching to producing other products, for example. With every decision, something 'has to give'. In the early days of mass production, the obvious place for this 'give' was the customer. So keen were customers to get their hands on products that they would be prepared to wait and wait and accept what were generally poor levels of quality – they knew no different.

'You can have any colour you like, as long as it's black.'
Henry Ford – talking of the Ford Model 'T'

Manufacturers had grown used to being the experts in what they do. The attitude of many manufacturers was that 'Customers should be grateful that we take the trouble to produce products at all'.

As markets matured and customer demands grew, the focus of control of processes began to shift. Whilst manufacturers had initially produced their products using their process, in effect producing what they chose to produce in the ways they chose, this began to change. Customers were no longer content to simply take what the manufacturer was prepared to produce and began to demand new products and services. Champions such as the JD Powers car surveys provided visible focal points, but in many other less public ways the discriminating customer began to place their demands on manufacturers.

Manufacturers would begin to learn that the needs of customers were taking an ever more important role in the way their business worked. They would come to learn that responding to these needs would not be a one-off switch in approach; rather it would be a continuous process of tracking changing customer needs and constantly refining approaches.

At first, with increasing supply, customers were able to start to make choices about the type of product they wanted to purchase and when. No longer could manufacturers afford the time to make products 'to order' as customers grew to expect to purchase items from stock. If your product was not available, they would find a competitor's that was. Thus manufacturers began to develop manufacturing approaches that ensured that their products were available and waiting for purchase.

Most manufacturers accepted that if their customers want next-day service (or anything like it), they'd have to buy the products 'off the shelf'. We can't make them that quickly, so we'll have to build up some stocks. The customer gets what they want when they want it, and our job is to replenish the stocks before they run out. We'll be 'buffered' against the uncertainty of the demand, and will be able to make things in nice, big batches ('Economic Order Quantities') so that once a machine has been set up to do something particular, it can keep doing it for a long time before it has to stop to be set up for something else. Thus manufacturers were able to meet the changing demands of their customers.

As mentioned above, these changes were part of a balancing act, and the something that had to give was the cost. Of course, all that extra material that has to be stored, as finished goods and as half-finished products queuing up for the next process, takes up space. And space costs money. So does the 5% (or so) of extra material that was often processed every time, to cover for the wastage that habitually occurred somewhere between the raw material and the finished product. But it'll be worth it if the job gets done and the customer gets what they want, and it's the only way of achieving this.

Or is it?

Some manufacturers recognised these shortcomings and saw the chance for improvement in addressing them. They recognised the benefits that had been achieved but began looking for the next steps on the change journey. They began to discover and create new advances. In the rest of this chapter, we'll explore some of the advances that have been made, and some of the approaches that have delivered them.

Pull don't push – a response to the challenges of scale, complexity and loss of control

Making a single product in small numbers is simple, but quite limiting in terms of commercial success. Manufacturers have tended to drive up the scale of their operations in order to achieve market share and economies of scale, and to offer multiple products so that customers have choices. The consequences within the factory can be quite challenging:

- different products follow different routes through the various production processes; scheduling, troubleshooting and progress chasing become onerous and endless tasks
- machinery which is heavily used during the production of one product isn't needed at all for another.
- people, who could cope easily with the demands on their time imposed by 50 per day of product A, find that they are over-stretched when the pattern shifts to 20 As, 20 Bs and 10 Cs.
- production quantities are rarely stable; just when we seem to have settled into a steady state, something happens in the market place and suddenly we need to double the production rates of one product and halve the rates of another.
- all in all, managers experience a loss of the feeling of being in control.

A natural and widespread response has been to introduce systems which attempt to plan, monitor and control responses to these challenges of scale and complexity. The second half of the

20th century saw the creation and evolution of several species of increasingly elaborate manufacturing, planning and control systems, which consumed the manager's assumptions, forecasts and knowledge, and returned instructions to follow for optimum results, and predictions of what those results would be. Rules were built into these models – rules that would ensure that the maximum number of customers would wait the shortest possible time for the products they were keen to obtain; and rules that would enable managers to extract the maximum possible value from every minute of every day in terms of the utilisation of their human and technological resources.

There have been high hopes for such systems since they first began to emerge, and in some ways they have delivered what they promised. However, each new generation of system has failed to deliver the comprehensive solution that its inventors have aimed for. None has proved to be the panacea its users have sought. Some manufacturers have achieved outstanding performance to which their planning and control systems have no doubt contributed; but most have found that their inability to achieve the balance and control they craved has, if anything, got worse as time has passed.

Why is this? Well, if we knew all of the answers to that question, we'd be rich and retired, but part of the answer is by now well known. It seems to have first occurred to a senior manager of a manufacturing company when he was walking around a supermarket. It struck him that the challenge of keeping the shelves stocked with just the right amounts of merchandise, despite the variability of customers' demands, had similarities to some of the challenges of running his car plant. From that thought grew the approach that became known as 'pull production', and the realisation that all that elaborate effort to 'plan and control' production facilities was founded on a set of false assumptions. The attempt to predict and control the complexity of a production facility, at ever-increasing levels of detail, was doomed to failure. 'The system' was *pushing* material into the front end of a complex set of processes on the basis of an imperfect model of those processes that could never be perfected. Every time the practice varied from the theory (which was inevitably happening almost everywhere, almost all the time), the net result was *waste*. Waste in the form of unnecessary delay; waste in the form of backlogs and queues, and unnecessary consumption of expensive space and time and other resources; waste in the form of unfulfilled promises and dissatisfied customers; and, in a vicious circle, waste in the form of 'underground action' by various players in the system who sought

[i] Monden Y, *Toyota Production System: Practical Approach to Production Management*, Industrial Engineering and Management Press, Norcross, Georgia, 1983.

[ii] Schonberger RJ, *World Class Manufacturing: the Lessons of Simplicity Applied*, The Free Press, New York, 1986.

[iii] Cheng TCE, Podolsky S, *Just-in-Time Manufacturing: an Introduction*, Chapman and Hall, London, 1993.

[iv] Womack JP, Jones DT, *Lean Thinking: Banish Waste and Create Wealth in your Corporation*, Touchstone Books, London, 1998.

[v] Slack N, Chambers S, Harland C, Harrison A, Johnston R, *Operations Management*, Pitman Publishing, London, 1995, pp. 628–629.

to buffer themselves and their interests against the other wastes, and ended up inadvertently only magnifying their effects and exacerbating the problems.

The flash of inspiration was that a change of mindset was needed, to switch the emphasis from *push* to *pull*. The basis of a supermarket's approach is that once enough people have taken six-packs of strawberry yoghurt from the cool shelf and through the checkout, a 'trigger' is activated which sends a signal to the store-room and *pulls* more yoghurts onto the shelf. Once the stock level in the storeroom falls to a pre-determined level, another signal is sent from the storeroom to the previous link in the logistics chain that brings the yoghurts from the factory to the supermarket – i.e. the storeroom *pulls* more yoghurts through the pipeline *as they are needed*. The storeroom on the supermarket site is relatively small – it has to be – and if it was replenished on a *push* basis, it would overflow as soon as the demand for a few items differed from the forecast (which happens all the time – the only thing we really know about forecasts is that they are almost never exactly right!). Supermarkets have this pull approach off to a fine art, and it has been that way for years. And since the 1980s, many (but by no means all) manufacturers have switched the emphasis of their materials control from push to pull, and achieved dramatic improvements in their ability to make and deliver the products that customers want, when they want them. All sorts of benefits follow, including some surprising ones like improvements in quality and in staff morale. We won't go into all the details here of the specific techniques that are applied to enact the *pull* approach, both within individual businesses and throughout entire 'value chains', but if you're interested then read up on subjects like 'Just in Time manufacturing', 'Pull Production' and 'Lean Thinking' – the 'business section' of the library shelves are full of books on these subjects, and some examples[i,ii,iii,iv] are listed, including one example[v] of the direct application of 'Just in Time' techniques in a health care setting.

Let's look at some more examples of advances achieved in manufacturing in recent years, to illustrate other steps in the production change journey.

Supplier development

If we think about the pull approach outlined above we can see that it creates the opportunity and the need for changes in supplier relationships. In the push approach, manufacturers have elaborate, albeit inaccurate, plans for future production. These plans set out, for example, the numbers of parts to be purchased from suppliers. Each of these parts has a cost and a great deal of effort is expended in trying to drive down these clearly identifiable costs. The approach taken is characterised by the creation of a competitive market in which the manufacturer sets potential suppliers against each other, with the constant threat that failure to deliver at reduced cost will lead to a change of supplier. The relationship between manufacturer and supplier is therefore potentially highly confrontational with much effort expended on contractual issues and a consequently very guarded relationship. This may have some success in driving down the unit costs of supplied components, but creates an environment in which there is little sharing of aims and ideas that may form part of an improvement approach. The relationship lacks trust and is denied the openness and freedom of thinking and sharing that are required to respond to change; to create agility. We have seen that agility requires an ability to question, understand, challenge and change. An environment of threats and fear is unlikely to foster this ability.

Manufacturing organisations began to review the balance of this approach, offsetting the focus on short-term financial savings of unit cost, with the ability to operate in a responsive and agile way. As they began to see the benefits of applying the pull approach within their organisations, it became clear that the improvements gained could be magnified if this pull were extended through their supplier base. In our supermarket example above, this creates a chain of triggers that extend back through the supply chain allowing the benefits to be felt by all, rather than the supermarket simply shifting its supply problem onto the shoulders of its suppliers.

To gain these benefits the relationship between purchaser and supplier, throughout this chain, has to change. At the outset organisations clearly need to communicate and share information, to allow the basic supply mechanism to work. Beyond this, leading organisations began to see that there were benefits in sharing much more than this simple day-to-day operational data. In order to stay ahead, manufacturers recognised that they relied not just on the quality of today's parts supplied by their suppliers, but on knowing that their suppliers were developing tomorrow's parts that they could incorporate in their future products. The manufacturers of products that you and I buy on the High Street, began to share their aims and plans with the suppliers of the parts and materials they use to make these products. This provided them with insights into where they saw their business going in ten years time so that they could align, where appropriate, their strategic and operational plans. Far from the adversarial environment of the push approach, they began to create real partnerships, in which not just aims were shared, but resources, funding, research and development and manufacturing facilities. In many of these organisations teams of workers from suppliers work alongside members of their customer organisation in fully integrated teams and are largely indiscernible from the organisation's employees.

The latest description of this development of organisations is termed the virtual organisation. This term captures the concepts that the definition and boundaries of an organisation which traditionally may have been the perimeter fence, or the employee roll, are being replaced by a much more flexible, shall we say agile, picture in which the nature of an organisation is constantly changing to meet the needs placed on it. The organisation moves from being a fixed facility looking for things to apply itself to, to becoming an agile capability seeking to respond to needs.

The move to Virtual Organisations is itself an excellent example of how changes create the opportunity for further changes where organisations are open and responsive to these opportunities.

There are a number of other areas that you may wish to explore, if the change bug begins to bite. Many of these are simple ideas, particularly when viewed with hindsight, but none the less powerful for that. Often, despite their simplicity, they were learned through painful experience that it would be a tragedy to have to repeat.

Fool-proofing techniques

This is a really simple idea, founded on the belief that, 'if it can go wrong, it will go wrong'. Fool-proofing is a slight misnomer in that it sounds like it is protection against fools. What it does in reality is provide protection from human nature by seeking to prevent an error from taking place, even though the chances of that error may be very rare, and other checks and safeguards may be in place. Fool-proofing is particularly important when applied to situations where an error can have very serious consequences.

Human nature of itself is a very valuable element of agility. The fact that we don't always do things the same way, or even always do the right things, is a powerful source of change opportunities, and can often lead to new discoveries. It is, however, a source of danger if the actions required to be undertaken rely upon being followed precisely for safety.

Sadly it appears that in order to respond to the danger presented by such circumstances, we require a real disaster before we act. As humans we often miss the opportunity to correct a problem when presented with a warning.

A particularly poignant example of fool-proofing is the death of Roy Chadwick who was a leading aircraft designer. He was responsible for the design of the Lancaster bomber famed for its exploits in the Second World War and the initial design work on the four jet Vulcan bomber which provided a major deterrent force in the cold war. In addition to many other projects, he was designer of the Avro Tudor four engine passenger plane. In 1947 he was to die in the crash of the Avro Tudor II prototype aircraft. The aircraft had undergone some routine maintenance, during which the aileron controls were disconnected. The ailerons are control surfaces on the wings of the aircraft that allow the pilot to control the roll of the aircraft by transferring his movement of the control wheel through cables to the ailerons. Unfortunately when these were reconnected the cables were reversed. Following appropriate procedures the work was checked by the maintenance crew, inspected and approved and, with the error undetected, the aircraft panels replaced. All was not lost, however, as the pilot will routinely check control movement before take-off with confirmation that the controls have full and free movement by an observer on the ground. Unfortunately this confirmed the controls moved when directed, but not that they actually moved in the opposite sense. When the pilot commanded them for a roll to the left, they actually moved in the opposite sense to roll the aircraft to the right. Checks completed, the aircraft was signalled OK for take off and its fate and that of those on board was cast. As the aircraft lifted off, the slightest roll of the aircraft due to wind was 'corrected' by the pilot but actually caused the roll to increase, rapidly leading to greater correction and an inevitable crash.

That such a brilliant designer should be lost in such a simple accident was a tragedy. There were checks in place, and they were carried out. How many times these checks had been completed on other aircraft and had saved the aircraft from certain disaster, one can only guess. With each occurrence an aircraft had been saved, but the underlying problem had not been removed. What hadn't happened, and would now, was the simple remedy of making the connections between the two sets of cables non-interchangeable. Thus 'fool-proofing' the possibility of this error occurring was removed. This was a simple, straightforward remedy that took no great creativity and added little if any cost.

There are many, many similar examples to illustrate the need for fool-proofing and our tendency not to see it until it casts a shadow.

A relative of fool-proofing is failsafe. Again a simple idea, this time founded on the belief that everything will go wrong, and when it does, one needs to minimise the failure to have as safe a condition as possible.

Again there are many examples but a graphic and easily understood one is the use of semaphore signals for the railways. At the outset of railway development, semaphore signals were used to indicate whether it was safe for a train to proceed. The signals basically comprised an arm which could be raised or lowered and signalled to the train driver the state of the track ahead. The original design held the arm in the safe position, and was moved to indicate danger. Now you may guess that there might be many reasons why the arm could be prevented from moving, ice being one of them and we have a system just waiting for a disaster to happen, and they did before the design introduced the simple change of making the signal rest in the danger position. An obvious solution but one that was only introduced following fatal accidents.

Another example, from the development of the railways, is the continuous braking system; a feature of all passenger trains for many years. These brakes rely on low pressure vacuum to release the brakes applied to every wheel of the train. Vacuum supplied by the engine releases the brakes; loss of vacuum through fault of any kind causes immediate application of the brakes bringing the train to a rapid halt. The 'fail safe' in this case is a stopped train. A simple system, and perhaps obvious, but it took the deaths of 25 people in two separate accidents where carriages had become detached from their engines to spur the development and use of this simple fail safe device.

In conclusion

We are not attempting to offer a catalogue of things that have been done or things to do. Our aim is to illustrate that there is much hard-earned experience that may be of value to organisations and people who have recognised the need to improve and are open to sharing and learning.

Space prevents us from exploring in depth the many other examples and other facets of how 'reducing work in progress and waste' has been a key focus of some dramatic improvements in leading manufacturing businesses in recent years. The thinking has been developed further in some ways under the guise of the 'Theory of Constraints'[vi,vii] and 'Agile Manufacturing',[viii] and these ideas are worthy of further investigation for those whose imagination is fired by the ideas discussed in this chapter. Hopefully the point is made – that these ideas, and the thinking behind them, might have something significant to offer those, like yourself, who seek to break the mould of some of the traditional thinking that constrains the performance of parts of our health care systems.

As these brief glimpses into different worlds have shown, progress takes the form of a journey where each step builds on those that precede it and creates the platform for those that will follow. Agility begins with the recognition that this is the nature of change and thrives where organisations embrace the process of challenging, learning and improving what they do and achieve.

The journey for production organisations moves on as customers place new demands and the most agile organisations succeed in meeting them. As an example, in what we now term the information age, customers are no longer content with simply placing orders and receiving products. They want to get inside the production facility, influence designs, follow the progress of manufacture and track the delivery in ways that were both impossible and undreamed of a handful of years ago.

There are parallels here with the changing demands and expectations being placed on health care organisations. Here too, the journey continues.

[vi] Goldratt EM, Cox J, *The Goal*, Gower, Aldershot, 1984.

[vii] Goldratt EM, *What is This Thing Called Theory of Constraints and How Should it be Implemented?* Croton-on-Hudson, N.Y.: North River Press, 1990

[viii] Dove R, 'Knowledge management, response ability, and the agile enterprise', *Journal of Knowledge Management*, 3(1), 1999, pp. 18–35

5 | Using stock, flow and trigger (SiFT) mapping to visualise, analyse and improve systems

Sarah W. Fraser, Penny Shuttleworth

Overview

Health and social care is organised in complex ways, and much of the care that is provided for patients and users, and the decision processes along the way, is tacit – it can't easily be seen. One of the fundamental practices in improvement methodologies is to map the processes under investigation so the activities, tasks and decision points can more easily be recognised. Once acknowledged, teams can discuss how best to make changes that will deliver improved services.

In the National Health Service (NHS) there is a strong heritage of using these workflow-mapping techniques as part of the improvement process. Most project teams have found them a useful means of understanding what currently happens as well as finding new ways to redesign the process.[i] These techniques work best where the process has a clear start and end point, and proceeds in a fairly linear fashion. Whilst this tends to be the case when focusing on hospital or referral process, there are many improvement teams who are faced with a more complex web of interactions between individuals, and these linear workflow techniques have been found to be limiting, and at times unhelpful. For example, in the case of older people, they all have their own care pathway and it differs for each person, as they often experience multiple pathologies and complex social needs.

[i] Locock L, *Maps and Journeys; Redesign in the NHS*, HSMC Birmingham, 2001.

Acknowledgements

The OPSC project was funded by the NHS Trent Regional Office, led by Linda Tully. In addition, SiFT mapping was also piloted by the NHS London Region, with two of their teams participating in the London Older People Services Collaborative.

ii Fraser SW, *The Patient's Journey; 35 Tools for Mapping, Analysing and Improving Health care Processes*, Kingsham Press, Chichester, UK, 2002.

This chapter introduces you to the technique of stock, flow and trigger (SiFT) mapping. It is designed to support the improvement process for teams whose topics require investigation of how patients and users move around their system, but where there are no obvious pathways or where the number of options is significant. *Stock* and *flow* are concepts borrowed from the discipline of systems dynamics, and the concept of *trigger* is a new one, designed for and used by teams working on systems related improvement projects in the NHS.

Throughout this chapter, the theory is grounded in case study examples from the North Derbyshire team involved in the Older People Services Collaborative (OPSC) run by NHS Trent Region in 2001/02. This programme aimed to improve the timeliness and manner in which older people were moved around local systems of health and social care. The twelve locality teams represented health and social care agencies, primary and secondary care, clinical and managerial staff. The focus was on the whole of the local community; how the individuals, teams and organisations could better work together for the benefit of older people. At the first workshop, all teams participated in a SiFT process, drawing maps of their local system for older people transfers. Some teams went on to use these maps for further review and design work.

Mapping is a crucial activity in the improvement process

A map is a visual representation of features; it highlights the main characteristics of the system, showing how pieces are connected and can show how the patients move between points.[ii] It provides the reader with an overview of the 'whole' and a sense of its complexity. They can see the broader view of the system within which they are operating and it helps them identify the part they personally play in caring for patients and users.

A draft map provides an instant impression of the system and raises questions. Is it well organised? Are the movements and activities clear? Do we know where older people get transferred to and from?

The process of mapping is also important, as it is an opportunity for team members to discuss and debate issues, as they are made more transparent. Many are surprised at the complexity of what they thought was a simple system, and how little they knew about what actually went on. Most of the OPSC teams reported that they were taken aback at the number of places older people

Box 4: Case study 2 (North Derbyshire)

The drawing of the map started with initial confusion. What is she talking about? However a clear explanation at the start is important. For some reason I still have the notes written at that talk. We had aide memoire notes which said – STOCKS – capacity, utilisation, place, resources, constraints, elapsed and actual time and information. Well, we started with the basics i.e. the places where Older People were. We could have written much more if we had given examples of all the information and resources etc. We also had a note to remind us saying FLOWS – impact on capacity and demand, resources used, elapsed time and actual time. We kept referring to these. Very quickly the resources/stocks were drawn and there was lots of discussion about the flows. Even more cynicism about the flows and the limits on the flows and why they did or did not flow. From this we were asked to discuss triggers in and out. The idea of going to a hospital and pulling Older People out of them sounded bizarre, but then we thought more about it. Well what is Intermediate Care doing, nothing more than pulling Older People out of acute hospitals into facilities for intensive rehab. Home visits are a trigger out. It just seemed bizarre that something that takes weeks to carry out is seen to be a trigger.

Box 5: Doing the SiFT map

When we had finished the map, it just looked such a mess. It seemed to have comments written all over it. Then it was typed up which meant it was easier to see the stocks, flows and triggers. The map still looks like an extremely complex model. Yet, on one page, there is a map of the system, which covers health and social care for older people in North Derbyshire. It would take days of process mapping of different systems for the diverse organisations to produce something similar. The stocks, flows and triggers are not complete, it is the main features which were produced within the allotted time. These were the areas that the group felt were important.

Other people's maps looked equally complicated. Some groups included more primary care areas, housing and environmental issues. It was obvious that the systems were perceived differently in each locality.

It was helpful that the actual process of the drawing of the systems map was with people who worked at the coalface – who knew the frustrations and difficulties encountered during their work. It was done without the managerial excuses for the problems, and with a focus on exactly how they felt the system worked. It was very easy for the group to do, and it helped explain the system to those who did not routinely work in North Derbyshire.

iii Richmond B, 'Systems Thinking: Critical Thinking Skills for the 1990s and beyond'. *Systems Dynamics Review* 9(2), 113–133, 1993.

iv Womack JP, Jones DT, *Lean Thinking; Banish Waste and Create Wealth in Your Corporation*, Simon & Schuster: New York, 1996.

could be transferred between, and the messiness of the movements and connections. They agreed the short time they spent SiFT mapping helped them see their local system from a new perspective.

The systems imperative

Agile health care organisations are those that have not only streamlined and improved their processes, *but also* those who can operate and adapt at a systems level. Working with systems is far more than the often-used phrase 'whole systems approach' in health care – getting all the stakeholders in one room, hoping that involving everybody means it is a systems approach. Rather, it refers to those leaders and practitioners who can see patterns and not only events, and who look beyond the immediate symptoms to fix the root causes of problems.[iii] Agile leaders and team members are those who need to ensure their services continually adapt to the changing pressures from patients, management and government. Evolution of a service is where its own needs are met; on the other hand co-evolution is where leaders and practitioners constantly organise the delivery of care, taking others' needs into account as well as their own.

SiFT mapping is a technique to help develop systems thinking skills in health care leaders and practitioners. The explicit maps created helps the appreciation of the reflexiveness of systems; namely the way in which the parts interact and impact one another. Agile teams and organisations need to understand how their actions may affect others – for the better or worse. The analytical techniques also help to design processes where patients and users can be pulled through the system, instead of being pushed.[iv] This is a fundamental criterion for 'lean' processes and is a pre-requisite for agile systems.

Approaches to making systems more explicit

There are many different ways to make systems explicit through diagramming; SiFT is one of these and it draws on facets of others. SiFT is a non-pictorial method, though it could easily be supplemented with photographs or illustrations of the places involved.

Table 3: Categories and examples of non-pictorial diagrams

Classification	Structure and relationships	Temporally ordered
• Affinity diagrams • Matrices • Mind maps • Fishbone charts	• Organisational charts • Influence diagrams • Spray diagrams • Systems dynamics diagrams • SiFT maps	• Flow diagram • Activity sequence diagrams • Causal diagrams • Fishbone chart • Systems dynamics diagrams • Algorithms • Process maps • SiFT maps

Non-pictorial diagrams can be placed into three categories; *classification, structure and relationship,* and *temporally ordered.*[v] SiFT maps predominantly show the structure of a system, though they can also provide information about the order in which things happen (temporal).

Systems dynamics

Stock and flow modelling, that has its heritage in the field of systems dynamics as invented by J.W. Forrester in the 1960s, is a method for describing and simulating systems using computer programmes.[vi] Systems dynamics distinguishes between stocks and flows, and uses computing resources to simulate how the system changes and performs over time.

This is a very useful process. However, the majority of health care improvement teams have neither the technical expertise nor the time to carry out these sophisticated modelling techniques. The concepts of *stock* and *flow* used in SiFT have been taken from systems dynamics and used in a different way, without using computer programs or attempting to run large scale simulations.

The pragmatic approach to mapping systems

A SiFT map can be completed in an afternoon, though extra time for assessing the implications is always helpful. As one of the principles of improvement mapping is to enable participants to discuss and debate issues that arise, the process of the exercise is important. It is much easier if all the stakeholders in the system are represented, including patients and users.

[v] Robinson D, Hewitt T, Harris J (eds), *Managing Development; Understanding Inter-organizational Relationships,* Sage: London, 2000.

[vi] Forrester JW, *Industrial Dynamics,* MIT Press: Cambridge, 1961.

TO35314

The object of a SiFT mapping exercise is to create a diagram showing where patients and users gather (the *stocks*) in the system and then to connect these places showing how the patients and users move between them (the *flows*). *Triggers* are the reasons why the person moves from one place to another.

Stocks   Places where patients and users gather and accumulate e.g. home, hospital ward, nursing home, church or temple groups, hospice wards, primary care practice, family's home etc.

            This is shown on the SiFT map in a box – a rectangle or square. The name and details about the stock are written in the box

Flows   The direction and manner in which the patients and users move from one stock to another.

            This is shown on the SiFT map as a single-headed arrow (single-headed because a patient can't move in different directions at the same time). If the flow does reverse direction, then an additional arrow can be used.

Triggers   These are the reasons why the person starts to move from one stock to another.

            This is shown on the SiFT map by a circle which is at the point where the arrow (flow) leaves the box (stock). Trigger details are written inside the circle, or if there are too many, you can write them below the circle.

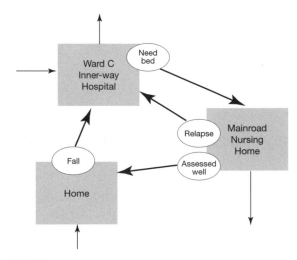

Figure 3: SiFT map

The SiFT map usually has around ten to twenty different stocks and a myriad of arrows connecting them. It looks messy (see the North Derbyshire Diagram).

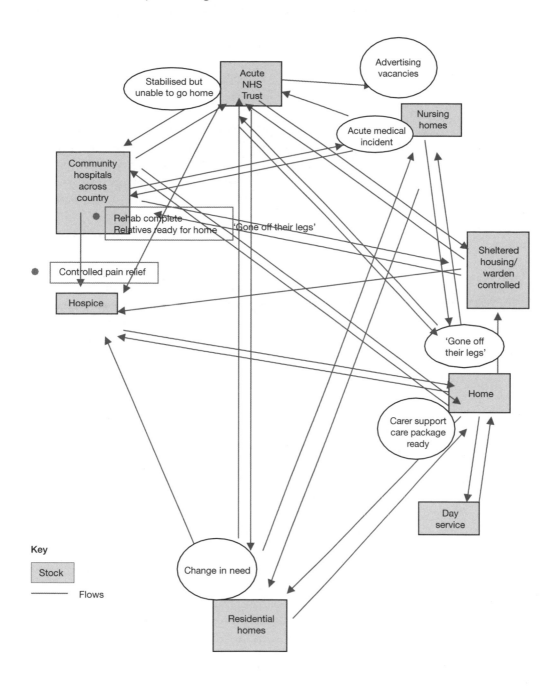

Figure 4: North Derbyshire – stocks and flows diagram
Care of the Older Person Collaborative Trent region

Facilitating the process

It is possible to produce a SiFT map in around two hours, though an afternoon allows for more time analysing and discovering ideas for improvement. The method below was the one used for taking the OPSC teams through their SiFT mapping process:

Preparation

Each team included representatives from a wide variety of stake-holders that had a common and explicit improvement objective. It helped by having more than one team as they could learn from each other. They agreed on the system to be mapped (how older people are transferred around their locality). The system needs to be one where there is a movement or flow of patients, equipment or information around a system. There is no need to define the system in great detail.

The teams had flipchart paper, Post-it™ notes, marker pens and pencils available. A five-minute creative warm up exercise was used to mark the changing of pace and style of thinking required for the SiFT mapping process. A facilitator led the teams through the activities. There was no need for the teams to be trained beforehand.

Identifying the stocks

After a brief description of what is meant by a stock, the teams were asked to brainstorm and identify as many as possible. They wrote the name of each stock on a Post-it™ note. Most of the OPSC teams came up with the following stocks: respite care, residential care, A&E, outpatient clinics, day hospital, GP surgery, X-ray department, community hospital, rehabilitation unit, private hospital, nursing home, medical assessment unit, rough sleepers (in doorways, parks), relative's home, hotels, religious and community support groups, and their own home.

It helped if teams named the specific hospitals, nursing homes and respite care facilities as this personalising of the map meant the process avoided becoming too theoretical.

Ordering the stocks

Teams were then asked to place their stocks (Post-it™ notes) on flipchart paper in any order. Some teams wanted to start organising the stocks and they were counselled to put the stocks anywhere, and to leave some room between each one so the flows (arrows) could be drawn.

One of the benefits of SiFT mapping is that is helps participants move away from the linear, step-by-step, pathway type thinking that they may be more used to, or prefer. Some teams found the apparent disorganisation and apparent messiness of SiFT mapping uncomfortable. They were reassured that there is no right or wrong way to produce a SiFT map and that the map will look chaotic – and that is fine.

Drawing the flows

The aim is to focus on the most common flows between the stocks. There will always be the exceptions and it usually isn't helpful to work on these at the first stage of a SiFT map. Teams were guided to use arrows to draw the flows that occur 80% of the time.

Most flows depicted the patient moving from place to place. However, it is possible to also include the information and equipment flows; in which case different coloured lines were helpful to distinguish between them.

Arrows cannot be double-headed so if there is a reverse flow, then an additional arrow needs to be drawn in. The purpose of separating these movements is to ensure that the reasons for the different directions in flow are discussed and analysed.

Analysing the stocks

With the project aims in mind, teams discussed issues arising from the map. For example, the North Derbyshire team discussed, as an initial basis, the areas where some members of the collaborative worked. The community hospital staff were soon drawing the links from where their patients came and to where they went. The care managers had a clear view of the stocks that were in the community. This led to a discussion of the problems of arranging care packages and the problems caused by funding. The issues were noted on the map.

Assessing the flows

The next step was to list characteristics of the flows. Usually there were three or four flows that seemed to be causing the most difficulty. Most teams started with these and then tried to capture something about every flow. For example the flows were often determined by means of transport and the delays caused by using different types of transport. We realised that one of the community hospitals had their own ambulance service that meant that patients flowed more smoothly and in a more timely manner to the next stock, whereas those waiting for the NHS ambulance service may have to wait in hospital for an extra day until an ambulance became available.

Prioritising areas for further investigation

At this stage the teams needed a little time to reflect on what they had produced so far. It was useful for them to articulate the surprises they felt, and the things that the map had raised that they hadn't thought of before.

The next steps involved looking at the triggers. Some teams met later and worked through all the triggers for all the stocks and flows. However, working on the key areas is usually sufficient to gain insight and learning into the system.

Teams were asked to identify the two or three stock-flow combinations that they would like to work with further. Some teams automatically chose the areas that they had always believed to be a problem, for example, the flow from hospital to patient's home (the discharge process). However, if they looked closely at their map, they could identify other areas that impacted on this stock-flow combination and felt it was worthwhile to work on them instead. For example, home to the accident and emergency department (A&E), or nursing home to A&E, were interesting stock-flow combinations to analyse as improvements that could improve the discharge process.

Assessing triggers

Based on the prioritised combinations, teams then identified what triggered the patient to move from one stock to another. The blunt end of each arrow is the point where the outward flowing trigger occurs. There may be more than one way to trigger movement.

For example, the care package being finally agreed is the most common trigger to move the patient from the hospital into residential care or back home. The trigger for someone to be admitted into hospital is often the diagnosis in A&E of 'off their legs'. This could be a medical reason but it can be a mixture of physical and social pressures that have led the GP to send them to hospital.

The trigger to a hospice from a community setting can be the inability to nurse the patient at home any longer or it could be for carers' respite or for pain control. Once the pain has been controlled, this could be the trigger to send them back to their originating place.

Ideas for improvement

Teams were then asked to gather ideas on how they could improve the whole of the system they were investigating. This meant looking for patterns and especially searching out where preventative action could avoid undesirable knock on consequences. The aim here was to produce ideas that went beyond traditional thinking and took the systemic nature of their issue into account. Some ideas that were captured in a few minutes at the OPSC workshop included: training carers, voucher system of access to health and social care, promoting independence of older people, focused health education, access to tests in different places, one-stop clinics, patient held records, single assessment etc.

Reversing the flow

As part of discovering ways to improve the system, teams worked on how they could reverse the flow of some of the arrows. For example, instead of the hospital pushing the patient out onto the nursing home, how could they find ways where the nursing home could pull the patient in towards them. For example, some nursing homes already send their matron to find out more about the patient. They also liaise with the care managers to tell them that they have vacant beds. In the SiFT mapping session, one of the ideas discussed was for nurses from the community hospitals going to the acute trust to see the patients who will be referred to them. It was thought this would improve the quality of the discharge and reduce the problems caused by the poor information flow between organisations.

Designing and planning

The final part of the mapping process was to agree on areas for further work, including where they felt a more traditional process map might be a useful exercise for some specific stock-flow combinations.

Benefits and limitations of SiFT mapping

SiFT mapping is best used for helping multi-disciplinary and multi-agency teams visualise and assess their system, to find common ground between themselves and to make the patterns in the system more explicit. The process enables team building, especially where different professions and organisations are seated around the same table. The broad overview nature of SiFT mapping and the way it is inclusive, requiring no definition of what is included or excluded, or where the process starts or ends, means it is easier and more collaborative an activity than doing a workflow map.

However, at some stage, teams will need to do some workflow mapping to get into the details of what they are changing. By relating this to the overview systems map, they should also be able to avoid making what appear to be quick wins, but in the long run make the situation worse for another stakeholder in the system.

Summary

SiFT mapping is a pragmatic technique for helping multi-professional and multi-agency teams to visualise the system they are working within. It is one way to stimulate discussion based on systems thinking rather than linear processes and procedures.

6 | Maximising the use of information systems

Nigel C. Bell, Sarah W. Fraser

Introduction

The delivery of high-quality health care is dependent on the deployment of high quality information systems; systems that are accurate, reliable, flexible and fit for purpose. These systems range from relatively simple transactional systems to complex decision support systems, from local systems to a national information infrastructure, and from specialised clinical applications to financial and administrative systems.

Transactional systems include applications like the electronic transfer of prescriptions between prescribers and dispensers, and the communication of pathology test requests and results. *Decision support systems* range from those used in general practice to inform prescribing decisions, to those used to assess the costs of particular health conditions and health care regimens for 'casemix' adjusted budget allocations.

Local systems include a wide range of home-grown and commercial systems in laboratories, general practices, and trusts. In the UK, the *national information infrastructure* includes systems such as the nationwide clearing service for administrative data on episodes of care, the national strategic tracing service for patient-identifying NHS numbers, and nationally managed but regionally delivered services for payroll, human resources, and financial management.

Specialised clinical applications include those that support specific conditions; often these support a specific care pathway for a specific condition in a specific organisational unit, but they may also be commercially available applications. *Financial and administrative systems* are necessary at all organisational levels, and as well as the nationally administered systems mentioned above there are systems for patient administration and for planning and budgeting at trust and health authority levels.

i Metes G, Gundry J, Bradish P. *Agile Networking*, Prentice Hall PTR, 1998.

As if the above dimensions do not themselves present enough of a challenge, the field of health care that these systems are trying to support is complex and ever-changing in terms of health care practices, pharmaceutical and surgical interventions, patient expectations, and of course organisational structures. The need for agility in information systems is both urgent and ongoing, not only in order to deliver information systems rapidly in order to bridge the presently huge gap between technical capability and the reality of deployment, but also to ensure that once those solutions are in place they are able to adapt quickly to a health care environment that is likely not only to continue to change but to do so increasingly quickly.

Finally, information systems do not only themselves need to be developed and deployed in an agile but responsive way; they also have the potential to support and enable greater agility in health care practice itself, proactively providing new opportunities for communication and decision-making. Rising patient expectations, new drugs and other interventions demand that health care practices and information systems establish a mutually respectful relationship in which systems respond to health care practice demands but also health care practices adapt to take full advantage of information system developments.

So what is the role of information systems in enabling and supporting agility in health care?

Earlier chapters in this book have presented a variety of definitions and explanations of the concept of 'agility'. In this chapter we will focus on four principles identified in *Agile Networking*[i] as:

- Enriching the customer
- Mastering change
- Leveraging resources
- Cooperating to compete.

Whilst these headlines have their appeal, we prefer to restate these as:

- *Listening to the outside* – continually monitoring an organisation's environment, particularly customers and competitors, and developing appropriate responses to its demands
- *Maintaining responsiveness* – maintaining organisational responsiveness at all levels and positively embracing change
- *Utilising all resources* – fully utilising all of an organisation's resources to respond and change

- *Extending capabilities* – extending an organisation's capabilities through partnerships and other alliances.

We will use this generic framework to look at the specific field of information systems in health care.

Information systems for agility

Listening to the outside

Whilst the language of 'customers and competitors' might sit rather more comfortably in the commercial world than in that of health care, health care organisations have as much need as their commercial counterparts to understand changing demands in order to shape appropriate responses. These demands come from patients, other providers, policy makers, and suppliers:

- *Patients* increasingly demand the same service levels they receive from commercial service providers – the health care equivalents, perhaps, of cash dispensers, 24-hour banking, internet banking, and booked appointments that fit their other commitments. They want increasingly to be involved in decisions about their own health care. And they want to receive excellent advice and excellent treatment, where necessary, with the latest technologies, techniques or drugs.

- *Other providers* raise expectations of what is possible, and provide valuable opportunities to learn from the successes (and failures) of others. These providers may be overseas or in the not-for-profit or private sectors of the UK.

- *Policy makers* determine overall health care priorities, set performance targets, and directly or indirectly determine financial allocations. The broadest definition of this group includes policy think tanks and the Royal Colleges.

- *Suppliers* seek to develop their own performance through offering innovative products and services such as analytical equipment, instruments, and pharmaceuticals. These can provide opportunities but can also raise expectations that become challenging demands.

Knowledge management is central to health care organisations' abilities to capture and disseminate knowledge of their operating environment. Internet technologies allow knowledge management (KM) solutions to be developed and deployed incrementally, using relatively simple components to build increasingly sophisticated KM capabilities. Intranets, for example, can move beyond telephone directories and newsletters to provide tools to support communities of interest around key topics, ensuring that information from outside the organisation is quickly assimilated, evaluated and used by those who find it most relevant.

It is widely appreciated, but nonetheless worth repeating, that KM is as much a cultural challenge as a technical one. Agility depends not only on capturing information but on getting it quickly and in digestible form to those who must make decisions based upon it. Rapid dissemination without rapid decision-making leads to information overload and a lack of responsiveness. Agility demands a degree of decentralisation in decision-making, and KM systems provide the information infrastructure that enables this.

Knowledge is about quality more than quantity. An often over-looked aspect of KM is dealing with the natural life cycle of knowledge, much of which degrades relatively quickly. Agility requires that knowledge is sometimes shared when it is incomplete; there are obvious risks with this, and lest there be any doubt, patient-specific information such as test results might be specifically excluded from such systems and practices, but to wait until all information is validated would deny an organisation its agility. The quality of, or confidence in, any information must be clearly communicated to all. It is also important that knowledge managers (or information owners) take responsibility for eliminating superseded, duplicated or redundant information if systems are not to become unusable.

Customer relationship management (CRM) systems have become something of a must-have fashion item in commercial and industrial sectors. The aim of these systems is to integrate customer information and transactions across the enterprise, making the customer's experience both more individual and more holistic. For example, an individual might interact with many departments of a telecommunications company – service plans and tariffs, bill payments and enquiries, equipment or service rental or purchase, fault reports, complaints, queries about the hole being dug outside one's house – and inadequate support from information systems can lead to a fragmented customer experience, with the need to repeat name and address and query details as the enquirer is passed from department to department.

In the Department of Health's semantics, an electronic patient record (EPR) describes in depth an episode of care and a health record (EHR) is less detailed but covers a much longer period, eventually from birth to death; CRM must accommodate both. Generic commercial solutions would need much tailoring in order to accommodate the intricacies of health care management, so it is likely that a degree of CRM functionality will be built into health record systems.

It is worthy of note that CRM is being paid much attention in UK local government, those frontline authorities with the unenviable task of joining up services provided by a huge diversity of central and not-so-central government departments so that these services can make some sort of sense to the recipients. Although health care is argued by many to not be a part of government, there are many areas where health care services becomes enmeshed with wider public service provision – road traffic accidents, drug dependencies, social services, and disability benefits are just a few examples.

To suggest that local authorities and health care organisations work together to develop common CRM solutions might be to over-constrain the problem by introducing too many variables; neither is it practicable to suggest that one waits for the other. But it is advisable for health care organisations to be aware of emerging cross-governmental and industry standards and practices, as sooner rather than later there will be an expectation that health care plays its rightful part in streamlined and integrated public service provision.

Maintaining responsiveness

For too many organisations, across all sectors, knowledge management has become knowledge collection – the amassing of large amounts of information for unspecified or forgotten purposes. From an agility perspective, organisations must be able to access this knowledge in meaningful ways in order to make informed decisions in order in turn to act appropriately.

Decision support systems draw together context-based knowledge and qualitative and quantitative information around key decision-making events. They support rather than replace recognised sources of expertise, and the most sophisticated will build the resulting decisions back into their knowledge bases in support of continuous organisational learning. Many health care decisions will continue to be based on years of personal and shared professional experience, and most of us would want it no other way, but where the event is relatively common, there can be significant value in having all the relevant supporting information to hand. Such events might range from basic protocols such as those of NHS Direct or support for prescribing decisions at the desktop to management decisions about investment and expenditure options.

Decision support systems have been around as commercial solutions for many years. Whilst there can be issues around technical integration with transactional systems, the bigger barriers to widespread implementation lie elsewhere.

Firstly, it can be a real challenge to identify not only the key decision points but also the relatively limited number of information items that play a *significant* role in the decision outcome.

Secondly, by definition such systems need to be tailored to the context of each organisation and this can be time-consuming and sometimes expensive.

Thirdly, there can be cultural barriers to accepting that a significant proportion of the decisions we make are relatively consistent and based on few parameters; we pride ourselves on our skill and judgement and dislike the thought that even a small part of this is relatively predictable and repeatable.

And finally, the design stage of decision support systems can highlight where decisions are *really* taken in organisations. For example, whilst a management board might formally sign off expenditure proposals, the reality is that in many cases the decision to spend how much with whom has virtually been taken by the person or team who prepared the expenditure request. Thus the information that informs the decision is of more use to other parts of the organisation than to the officially responsible decision maker. If senior management defensiveness kicks in, decision support systems can add little value as they map onto a formal power distribution rather than a real world one.

Agility requires clarity and commitment in all of the above – judgement over what information is important, realism about the scale of investment, and the maturity and courage to accept challenges to our expertise and authority. Decision support systems can support consistency in decision-making, but if an organisation is to be agile, decisions must be made at the lowest possible level in the organisation consistent with good governance. This in turn requires that authority, accountability and expertise are aligned, which is far more than a systems implementation challenge.

Intelligent software agents are at the leading edge of information technology. These are manifestations of complex adaptive systems in an information systems context, working in an information network that includes the internet and usually quite narrowly focused on a specific set of tasks. Agents, as their name implies, act on behalf of a user or a resource or a function, and communicate with other agents.

Typical applications include search facilities that use the network rather than sequential searching or indices, and resource allocation. An example of the latter of particular interest in health care might be the booking of consultant appointments. If we assume that it will be some time before a typical patient has an online agent-based diary system, then a starting point might be the provision by the patient of a list of possible dates and times for the appointment. A number of iterative conversations would then take place amongst agents representing both specialist consultants and the resources they need such as consulting rooms or specialist analytical equipment or operating theatres. A list of options could then be presented back to the patient.

Such intelligent software agents are ideally suited to complex environments in which change is frequent, as decisions are made on information that is as current as the nodes on the network. In traditional information systems, schedules of resources are typically centrally held, such as consultant's diaries, or might even be fixed or assumed, such as an operating theatre that is not already booked by another consultant; last minute changes to either may not always be reflected immediately in central schedules. By placing the agent close to the resource it represents, for example on the handheld computer of the consultant, currency of information is improved and, by conducting a network of conversations rather than an algorithmic calculation, scheduling performance is optimised. Some agents are even able to 'learn' from the usefulness of previous conversations, enhancing their performance further.

The theoretical benefits of agent-based information solutions are compelling in a number of scenarios. But the deployment of, and market for, such solutions is immature. Reasons for this include:

- **Architecture** – a lone agent is unable to converse. Existing applications would therefore need to be re-engineered to incorporate agent-based functionality. This must be done by the application developers rather than as after-market modifications by the implementer.

- **Market attractiveness** – agents themselves are relatively small and specialist applications, though the number of occurrences needs to be as large as the number of entities in dialogue (e.g. one per bed or one per patient). Current leaders in the application software market, such as Germany's SAP, provide large integrated application suites, so the model is quite different. The most likely route to market for those with the capability to develop agents is to work with these large providers rather than to market discrete agents

- **Standards** – in order to enter into meaningful conversations, agents need to be able to understand each other. Although a common language might be relatively easy to define within the confines of a single application or suite, standards must be agreed, developed and implemented if agents are to work across system boundaries

- **Stability** – all new technologies follow broadly the same life cycle, the early stages of which are marked by rapid development of multiple variations and biological-style adaptation and selection. Application developers will monitor, or participate in this stage of divergence and convergence with varying levels of interest, but all will be looking for the right time to commit in order to balance the risks inherent in doing so against the benefits of influencing the later stages of development.

In the search for information solutions to support increased responsiveness in rapidly changing environments, intelligent software agents appear very promising. But like many technologies before them, this promise will of itself be insufficient to assure a long and healthy future. Health service providers may wish to consider if and how to intervene in order to speed and facilitate this development and maturation process.

Utilising all resources

Given the right information from its environment, and having used this information to make the right decisions, how is an organisation to respond effectively? 'With all of the resources at its disposal' would be a worthy reply, but this requires a clear appreciation of what resources the organisation has and how they are currently being utilised.

In the previous section we saw the potential of intelligent software agents in helping to allocate resources through collaborative decision-making, and glimpsed some of the challenges that need to be met in order to see these technologies fully exploited. In the meantime, organisations must make use of the best available tools.

Enterprise Resource Planning (ERP) systems have their roots in a manufacturing environment, but can now be found in other sectors such as distribution and services, including health care. They tempt with the offer of the holy grail – comprehensive planning and performance management across all divisions and levels of the 'enterprise'. It is worth a brief detour into the world of manufacturing in order to better understand the principles and driving forces behind these widely deployed systems, and thence their limitations and some optimisation (or damage limitation) strategies.

The 1970s saw significant computer power starting to be deployed outside scientific applications. The first Material Requirements Planning systems took simple hierarchical Bills of Materials and used these to cascade demand for sub-components and raw materials for a specified number of end products. They generated work (production) orders from raw materials through sub-assembly to final product. The stimulus for production was often the falling of finished product stock levels to pre-determined 'safety' stock levels. These systems were to evolve in the late 1970s/early 1980s into more comprehensive Manufacturing Resource Planning (MRPII) systems that embraced features such as sales order processing, sales analysis, and sales forecasting, as well as more advanced features such as the handling of engineering changes (to ensure smooth transition to a new design, down to the level of a different bolt being accompanied by its requisite new nut!).

The 1980s saw much interest in the Japanese manufacturing management method of just-in-time. Manufacturers had traditionally sought efficiencies through long production runs or batch sizes, spreading the unit cost of the set-up phase for each product and generating large stocks to ensure supply until the next production run. As customers demanded greater variety and shorter lead times, these principles generated conflict between the demands of manufacturing efficiencies as analysed in unit costs and those of the market place as reflected in sales volumes. In just-in-time, stocks of raw materials and sub-components are minimised and batch sizes reduced, with the ultimate goal being a batch size of one. Three fundamental principles underpinning just-in-time are low stocks, flexible production, and 'pull' rather then 'push'. Low stocks minimise working capital and help avoid obsolete product stockpiles; flexible production units allow for quick changeover between products, reducing batch sizes and increasing variety; and production orders are initiated in response to known customer demand rather than by stocks falling to replenishment levels or by sales forecasts.

The limitations of traditional top-down planning and production techniques became more and more apparent and some of the major MRPII systems suppliers failed to respond effectively and went out of business. Increasing product variety, shorter product lifecycles, and increasing organisational size and complexity strengthened the need for comprehensive and sophisticated information systems, but by the 1990s the marketplace had become dominated by one supplier, the German company SAP, that offered a complex but highly configurable suite of applications that covered most of the activities of most production organisations. Implementation is expensive because of the degree of configuration possible (and necessary), but SAP is one of the success stories of the information systems industry.

Back in the complex world of health care, what can we learn from this, in particular when we seek to maximise the use of all our available resources in an agile way? Firstly, whilst ERP systems have a role to play, it must be more about ensuring that adequate resources are available for call-off than about top-down planning and control. Health care 'production units' must be given sufficient autonomy in decision-making if agility is to be sustained. This might mean, for example, that appointment bookings should be handled in a distributed manner, with decisions being taken at the point of maximum knowledge, rather than as a central administrative function. Information systems must be capable of being configured to reflect this.

Secondly, we usually deal with 'batch sizes' of one in health care. Whilst there are many routine operations performed almost in production line fashion, there are also many unique combinations of requirements. 'Your appointment will take place at this location on this date with consultant X' is not acceptable in a world of patient-centred health care. So multi-skilled health care practitioners, and multi-purpose equipment and consulting rooms and operating theatres must increasingly become the norm. The interface between ERP-style systems and, say, electronic health record systems must be constructed so that patient needs are a driving input to planning processes.

Finally, the concept of 'pull vs. push' has some important cultural aspects. One of the reasons why so many British and US manufacturers failed, or took a long time, to adopt just-in-time was that they tried to adopt some of the tools and techniques without adapting management cultures. Just-in-time cannot succeed in an environment of centralised control, a lack of real understanding and appreciation of customer needs, and a set of performance indicators that emphasise unit costs. Management reporting must often address a large number of externally dictated performance indicators, but care must be taken in ensuring that these do not encourage and reward behaviours and decisions that work against the needs of agility.

Organisational **intranets** have huge potential for maximising the effectiveness of the organisation's resources. Formal, structured decision-making, as described above, requires the support of extensive staff communications through a variety of channels, and intranets can be excellent contributors to this. But too many organisations stop far short of fully exploiting intranet technologies, held back by out-of-date hierarchical mindsets and a lack of vision about real staff engagement.

Too many intranets are little more than an on-line version of long-standing staff communication methods combined with hi-tech archiving. Newsletters, team briefings, management memoranda, operating procedures, staff notices, meeting minutes from months or years ago ... many organisations fail to provide even such basic facilities for two-way communication as suggestions schemes and letters pages.

The real power of the internet is its ability to connect large numbers of people with common interests and informal relationships – 'communities of interest'. Intranets are built on the same technology platforms, but rarely exploit their features in the same way. This is a major missed opportunity to fully utilise the organisation's most valuable resource – the energy and creativity of its people.

Alongside the formally structured relationships in organisations, we all know there are informal relationships that appear on no organisation chart – departmental football teams, cyclists, motorcyclists, charity supporters, golf enthusiasts, music lovers, gardeners, cooks. There are also those who share a work-related interest, perhaps trying to solve a problem or find creative ways around a difficulty. The internet supports such communities of interest not only with links to others but also with some more proactive services. 'Ask Jeeves' is an example, where acknowledged experts and informed amateurs contribute information and ideas relevant to a particular issue.

Organisations serious about maximising agility should consider how their intranets can help people to connect. There is little more powerful than a group of people who care about something working collaboratively, yet many organisations do not tap into this energy. The stimuli that require agile responsiveness are organisation-wide, not concentrated at senior management levels. Staff who can connect themselves in appropriate networks are able to bring tremendous energy to problem-solving. In adapting internet technologies for organisationally bounded purposes, many organisations have implemented old models of top down information flows and central editorial control. Serious consideration must be given to re-enabling some of the anarchy and diversity of the 'raw' internet in support of employee empowerment and organisational agility.

Extending capabilities

We have looked so far at how an organisation can use information systems to enhance its sensitivity to its environment, to enhance its responsiveness, and to use all of its resources in doing so. Our final theme is the extension of capabilities beyond the organisation's boundaries, in particular through partnership working.

Partnership working is first and foremost an issue of organisational leadership and culture; information systems aimed at fostering mutually beneficial relationships between organisations will fail or become redundant in an unsupportive cultural context. When senior management recognises the real benefits to patients of partnership working and commits the organisation to the necessary cultural change, demands are placed on processes and information systems to enable partnership working.

Partnership working requires changes in both structured and unstructured information flows. The former relate to transactional information flows, and are typically patient-related; examples include an ambulance service that uses information on bed availability to determine to which hospital a patient should be taken, or the transfer of a patient between general and specialist facilities, or between public and private health care providers. The latter relate to the sharing of intelligence, of contextual information, of anything that strengthens feelings of shared interests.

Extranet is the name given to intranets that have been extended beyond organisational boundaries. This is rarely done *in toto*, but specific areas of an organisation's knowledge base are opened to specific partners. Examples might include shared research or development interests, or issues of interest to organisations in geographical proximity. Some extranets, like intranets, do support business processes, and these can be extended across two or more organisations where the requisite levels of trust have been established.

Information standards continue to be a focal point for a great deal of activity and debate in the UK and international health care fields. Unfortunately for those dealing with real health care issues today, the promise often appears to be about a future perfect state when everyone communicates in a common 'language of health' that embraces technical standards, clinical terminology, and administrative data.

The realities of technological innovation and continuing developments in clinical practice mitigate against achieving long-term stability in information standards. It would be sensible therefore to identify a small number of critical data items and to use these in practice, adapting them in response to changes and extending to other data items in an evolutionary way; in fact, to apply the principles of agility to information standards development.

Where information standards are not formalised *and* put into universal use, organisations wishing to work in partnership with others will need to make pragmatic choices:

Firstly, it is important to be pragmatic. A local agreement on information standards that supports improvements in patient care today is valuable in its own right, whether or not it is entirely consistent with some yet-to-be-implemented formal standard. To borrow a phrase from environmental campaigners, 'Think global, act local'; awareness of developments at national and international levels is important but local action is where the real difference can be made, in this case to patient care. It is incumbent on the information systems and clinical coding functions within organisations to apply the principles of agility in this area, adapting and adopting standards as they become available, in a spirit of convergence.

Secondly, organisations should use what already exists. This might include technical standards such as the e-Government Interoperability Framework (eGIF), Clinical Terms ('Read codes') or SNOMED, or HL7. Despite the fact that most of these are in various stages of development, subsets have often been agreed and these can support information sharing in relevant technical or clinical areas. In the area of administrative data, even the use of national patient identifiers such as the NHS Number in England is not yet consistent, with too many organisations happy to rely on surname and postcode despite the danger to patients.

Thirdly, organisations should remind themselves of the Pareto principle; 80% of the benefit will arise from 20% of the activity in any given field. The phrase 'minimum data set' is much used, but in too many cases these have taken years to develop and have become maximum data sets. Clinicians are sometimes asked to collect huge numbers of data points, on the basis that management and administrative information should be drawn from operational data. This is a noble aim, but the impact can be that operational effectiveness is hampered by the burden of data collection for (often unspecified) future administrative use and analysis.

Concluding remarks

The capabilities of information systems seem often to be limited only by our imagination, yet so much of what we see and experience falls far short of this massive potential. Information systems are not sufficient to achieve organisational agility, and anyone launching an IS-dominated 'agility project' should expect little return on their substantial investment; yet to attempt to develop agility without exploiting information systems would be to do so without one of the most powerful tools available to organisations today.

This chapter has explored some key themes related to agility and information systems:

- The role of knowledge management and customer relationship management systems in helping organisations to listen to the outside;
- The challenges of exploiting enterprise resource planning systems and intranets in order to utilise all of an organisation's resources;
- The potential of decision support systems and the promise of intelligent software agents for maintaining responsiveness; and
- The use of extranets and information standards to extend an organisation's capabilities.

The field of information systems changes with breathtaking speed, so this necessarily selective assessment may have been different twelve months ago or may be different again in twelve months' time. A modest objective of such a snapshot might be to sow the seed of a conversation between IS managers and those leading organisational change, and if this chapter helps to make that a reality in only a handful of health care organisations, then it will have made a worthwhile contribution.

7 | Teaming and leading in an agile system

Maxine Conner

The purpose of this chapter is to help readers consider the nature of the team and the leader within the agile health care setting. The perspective is a personal one and reflects my own enquiry into the ideas and concepts of agility. This chapter represents personal observations, critical appraisal and ideas about how we might help our teams and leaders become more agile as they strive to deliver first class health care services.

[i] Stahr H, Bulman B, Stead M, *The Excellence Model in the Health Sector*, Chichester, UK, Kingsham Press, 2001.

The patient/health care practitioner interaction

The building block of health care is the interaction between the patient (or service user) and the health care practitioner. During this interaction the patient seeks support, guidance and expertise in helping them to solve a deeply personal and individual problem. Every health care practitioner reciprocates by investigating and probing the patient's individual context to design a diagnostic, treatment and support pathway which is both highly effective and satisfying to each individual patient. The ability to consistently deliver this interaction is the hallmark of the agile health system.

Agility in the health care context

If the hallmark of agility is the ability to deliver a highly satisfying and consistent patient pathway then the delivery mechanisms must also be agile. Stahr, Bulman and Stead[i] provide a simple framework that represents the health care delivery system.

ii Sharifi H, Zhang Z, Agile Manufacturing in Practice Application of a Methodology, *International Journal of Operations and Production Management*, 21(5/6), pp 772–794, 2001.

iii Dove R, Design Principles for Highly Adaptable Business Systems, With Tangible Manufacturing Examples, www.parshift.com, 1999

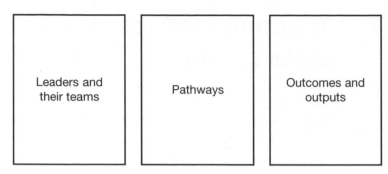

Figure 5: Schematisation of a care delivery system

Using this system, the interaction between the patient and the health care practitioner reflects a 'leader and team' context. It is to this contextual field that we must look to begin to understand the nature of agility.

So what does agility look like?

Having begun to explore the notion of agility it is intriguing to attempt to identify 'it' in clinical and management practice within the health care environment. Within the literature several ideas are frequently suggested to mean agile. Sharifi and Zhang[ii] describe the need to be able to change and adapt rapidly. In comparison, Rick Dove[iii] suggests agility is about the system having the competencies of being reusable, and easily reconfigurable to meet expectations as well as scalable to cope with changes in demand presented. What does all this mean?

Dove proposes that agile teams are 'response able', they are *able to respond* to ensure that their customers (patients) get the services they require. This clear and simple definition helps us observe and assess teams and leaders who appeared to be 'response able'. The observations here are purely subjective and are included as a way of helping readers new to the ideas presented in the book, to begin to think about the notion in relation to their everyday practice.

The agile team

Teams that exhibit exceptional levels of patient satisfaction, together with the ability to deliver clinical effective care, appear to demonstrate certain characteristics which make them 'response able':

Box 6: Team characteristics

- They constantly attune themselves to what their patients want
- They appear to prevent themselves from slipping into a paternalistic frame of mind which offers the patient what we 'the experts think is best'
- They constantly test their assumptions about what patients want and value, by engaging in a dialogue that is built upon a genuine desire to improve the patient experience
- They demonstrate an outstanding knowledge of what they actually achieve and know how to measure and monitor it
- They invariably know about teams who outperform them and are curious about how this improved performance is achieved
- They work in small cycles of planning, not more than 6 months and change their shape to fit what needs to be done
- They naturally project their work forward, by planning in a meaningful way, a way which is about action not prevarication.

Not only listening but anticipating

One characteristic that can be seen in agile teams is that of patient centredness. Such teams are not just focused on their patients, they are intrigued by them and they truly centre their work upon the needs of the patient. They are like a photographer with his subject in the viewfinder. They are conspiring to keep the patient in the viewfinder and continuously adjust to ensure they have a clear picture. This constant refocusing seems to be an important sensing device that helps the team to address the issue of adding the value that the patient wants. It appears to link to the characteristic of avoiding benign paternalism and it is this constant refocusing and centring on the patient that is perhaps the reason that they avoid the attitude that 'we know best'.

Agile teams also appear to go beyond the normal bounds of trying to satisfy patients. They listen constantly to ensure they can surpass the expressed needs of the people they serve. They appear to be able to anticipate what might delight the patient, often before the patient even thinks of it. This skill seems to be akin to the entrepreneur who intuitively knows which product to produce, to satisfy a market that has not yet even been invented.

Box 7: An example in practice

Having started with the usual round of organisation level patient satisfaction surveys, a Radiotherapy team became dissatisfied with the type of information the high level survey produced. It provided a great starting point; however it raised more questions rather than helping build solutions. The application of the high-level survey set off a series of initiatives which enabled the team to listen to, then anticipate, the needs of their patients. Moving on from the survey they introduced the following approaches to assist them in their quest for improvement:

- A specifically designed survey, asking the questions the primary survey helped them surface
- Patient feedback cards
- Telephone contacts to consider how improvements could have been made
- Focus groups to deal with specific issues
- A focus upon patient satisfaction during the routine delivery of care
- Extensive review of complaints at a departmental level.

Such tools may be viewed as facilitating the *response able* competency sought by an agile team.

At this point you may be thinking that you too have tried all of these things. However, the difference between an agile team and a traditional team is that the agile team will stick at such listening activities. They are more than just a passing phase; they are one of the cornerstones of their patient centredness. Furthermore, such teams also **do** something with the information they glean from all this activity. It does not 'sit on a shelf' gathering dust but is used to drive action and deliver improvement.

Standardisation to add greater value

Such agile teams have found out how to balance standardisation and customisation (or individualising) of the care process. They have buckled down and standardised what is important and controllable, they have effectively used the available evidence base and can usually produce their protocols, which are invariably up-to-date and used by all. They have a distinct competency of providing seamless and consistent technical care, which is perfectly routinised and satisfying to the patient. Mastering this part of the care process appears to free up both their time and the energy to reframe upon individualising the parts of the care pathway which the patients identify as important and make such a difference to the overall experience.

Insiders who can become outsiders

When I first began to consider high performing agile teams I began to see a feature which was common to many of them. They constantly benchmarked the patient experience to the technical and clinical scrutiny of their relevant professional standards. They practised at the level of the best, or usually somewhere near it. However they also did something else.

This feature tacitly performed was difficult to isolate and much time has been spent with many teams discussing their service provision before I fully appreciated its significance. Such agile teams also seem have the ability to think like the patient – they can turn themselves inside out. They measure service delivery not only from their own expert position, but from the perspective of 'is our service good enough for my family?'. This appears to provide an interesting set of triangulating perspectives.

This constant focusing and refocusing using the different perspectives and the intelligence and know how from each one, appears to be key to the idea of a 'response able' agile team. Their ability to respond in an agile manner comes from the different views they take of the patient experience; they are not stuck and

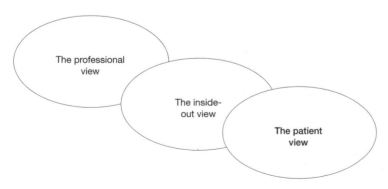

Figure 6: A triangulation of perspectives

do not suffer group think, they constantly push back the boundaries of what is possible.

Performance managers at the level of service delivery

How do agile teams become so agile? One of the key issues seems to be that they know more about their work than anyone else. You may argue that teams always do; however agile teams have a command and grasp of the data which are a part of their service delivery mechanism. They recognise that the level of aggregation of data undertaken within the NHS makes the data useless in terms of helping a team improve. Data are usually aggregated to the level of a functional service and not at the level of the patient pathway.

Agile teams recognise this fact and actively seek to improve the data they have. They do not wait for the health care system to provide them with the data they need. They create the data often in spite of the system. An often repeated story describes how the team had to start from scratch, manually collecting the data they knew to be important, with few if any people in the system recognising and supporting their endeavour. The people in the team truly and effectively manage their own performance.

Box 8: An example in practice

What do you need to measure to understand your service, and equip yourself to become response able? Experience with over 200 teams suggests that some of the teams striving to become more agile and response able need to ask themselves the following critical questions:

- How many patients come through your system each day, week, month and year?
- How has this changed over the past three years?
- How long does the overall patient journey take?
- How long does each step of the journey take?
- Where are the bottlenecks that limit the patient's ability to move smoothly through the system?
- What value does each step bring to the patient?
- How satisfied overall are the patients?
- Which step do they find most dissatisfying?
- How clinically effective is the overall care process?

Leading the agile service

Having identified that agile teams are *response able* teams, the final part of the chapter aims to helps you consider the function of the leader or leaders in such a team. Although the hierarchy continues as an organisational form bringing with it control and centralisation, only rarely if ever does one discover a team with only one leader. Many teams that provide health care services are geographically dispersed and are full of leaders working in both formal and informal leadership roles. At times within the complex environment of health care we all take the lead, but at other times we follow the lead of others. Effective leaders in an agile system know how to do both, and do so at the right time.

Alignment is critical

Within an agile system the leader focuses upon the needs of the people, as the people centre on the needs of the patient. This feature is not unique to the agile leader but appears to be dominant in such teams. The leader ensures that the work environment is supportive to the development of each and every individual working to deliver the service.

However, focusing solely upon the needs of the staff is insufficient to deliver the response ability teams are seeking. The leader of the agile team seeks continuously to balance and align the multiple agenda of all the people and organisations who are involved in the service delivery.

When you first attempt to consider the multitude of objectives involved in system-wide service delivery, it often seems that some objectives are contradictory. Often they are; the trick here is not to focus on which is most important but to attempt to identify which ones are complementary.

As individuals, teams and organisations work collaboratively on issues they are all united in; they build the relationships that will be the base from which they move forward onto the more contradictory objectives.

Traditionally we have all fallen into the trap of thinking that we must select which is most important. The agile leader will find a way of recognising what is common between all the seemingly competing agendas, and align what is common and purposeful. The leader recognises this pattern and the value in the 'easy' stuff, and creates the space for people to learn to work together. This act of alignment, recognition and separation of contradictory work

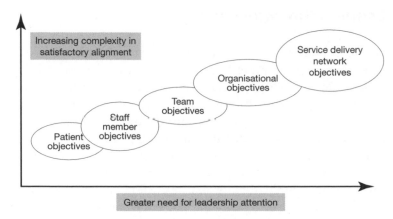

Figure 7: Leadership focus

can open up the debate about how the objectives can be achieved and also builds the working patterns of how the solutions may be found.

Getting started

Developing the key competencies associated with agility can appear complex but in fact starting with what you already do well will assist any team to speed up their ability. Key areas for action are:

Table 4: A starting point for thinking about agility

	Key area	Preliminary action which can be taken
1.	Understanding what patients actually want	• Dig out the old surveys of patient satisfaction • Revisit them to learn from them, consider how much action was taken. • Build up an approach to collecting information from patients, use lots of approaches, small-scale data collection and act on it.
2.	Understand what you currently achieve	• As a team, spend time thinking about what you achieve, starting anecdotally, but then critically appraising what you actually know about the performance of your service.
3.	Understand who, where and how teams outperform you	• Seek out practice that is better than yours – continuously. • Meet with such teams, spend time understanding how and why their results are different. • Bring back some ideas and design them into your approach. • Use short cycles of change, which can be reversed if the change is not effective.
4.	Understand what stops you from responding fast and flexibility	• Thinking through the factors that currently limit your flexibility is critical. • Working out an action plan to remove or get round the blockages will be critical. • Being bold enough to put your plan into action.

8 | The journey to agility: case studies for improving the care of older adults in London

Val Jones, Amanda Layton, Jean Andrews, Ruth Adam, Alan Beaton, Keith Strahan, Sarah W. Fraser

Background

The London Older People's Service Development Programme is an innovative two-year programme whose goal is to promote independence among London's older people through delivery of person-centred, coordinated services. Commissioned in December 2000 as a means of pulling together three policy strands – older people's services, the NHS modernisation agenda and primary and community care development – it capitalises on the success of the collaborative improvement methodology (see overleaf) in other 'modernising' initiatives in the National Health Service – cancer and coronary heart disease, for example.

Working across health and social care, and focusing on introduction of the single assessment process, the programme makes a significant contribution to the NHS Modernisation agenda, helping to implement the National Service Framework for Older People and bringing fresh ideas to service planning and development. With a strong focus on prevention and adopting a whole systems approach to service redesign, the programme is achieving success in improving the experience of care for older people and strengthening partnership working across the capital. *Right care, right time, right place* are the watchwords.

Acknowledgement
The project work for these case studies was funded by the former NHS London Regional Office, (now Directorate of Health and Social Care, London) as part of the London Older People's Service Development Programme. These case studies represent some of the innovative work taking place, all resulting from the energy, enthusiasm and commitment of the teams involved.

[i] Institute for Health care Improvement, Boston, Mass, 1995 www.ihi.org

Each project is London borough-based and must include partners from primary health care and social services as a minimum; in practice, many also include partners from the acute, community, mental health and voluntary sectors. The first 13 projects began their work in November 2001, joined in May 2002 by a further 13, working either on 'case finding' of older people at risk of functional decline, or intensive 'case management' of high resource users. Some are focusing on falls; one is looking at early detection of dementia.

Falls represent a leading cause of mortality due to injury in people aged 75+. Two thirds of general and acute hospital beds are occupied by people aged 65+ and with social services spending on people in the same age group running at nearly 50% of their budgets, there has never been a better time to implement a programme which has prevention and the active promotion of independence for older people at its heart.

Collaborative improvement methodology

The 'collaborative' model is an improvement method developed by the Institute for Health care Improvement[i] in the USA and is now used internationally. It relies on the spread and adaptation of *existing* knowledge to multiple settings to accomplish a common aim. In the UK the methodology has been used in a variety of health care settings to improve services and patient outcomes; for example, reduction of waiting times for appointments in primary care, improving cancer services and improving recruitment and retention. The older people's programme has adapted this model to be effective across 'whole systems' of health and social care.

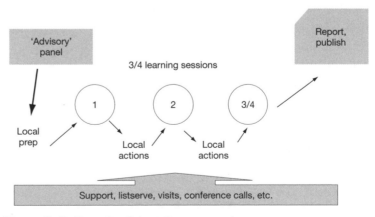

Figure 8: Outline of collaborative approach

Highly structured time limited programmes, involving many teams working to a common goal, 'collaboratives' offer a rapid, validated way of effecting service change and improvement. By utilising Plan, Do, Study, Act (PDSA) cycles to test small changes, teams working in collaboratives are able rapidly to spread successful outcomes and learn from what does not work well. During the programme, teams meet at a number of learning sessions to share good practice. In between these learning sessions they test and implement new ways of working using key change concepts (general notions or approaches to change that have been found to be useful). There is a strong emphasis on measurement and teams report monthly, both centrally and to each other, on their progress.

The momentum for change occurs through regular learning sessions, monthly reporting and an element of healthy competition between the teams. It is not a method for researching new knowledge, an easy fix, or a cheap option. At its inception the Development Programme did not consciously adopt the notion of agility as a means by which its projects would plan and progress their work. However, our experience, as described in the case studies, readily demonstrates that the concepts are a valuable tool for tracking progress, reviewing lessons learned and highlighting success and can be simply applied in a range of settings.

[ii] Maskell B, 'The Journey to Agile Manufacturing', www.maskell.com

Method for assessing progress and documenting case studies

As agility is still a contested concept for health care (see earlier chapters in this book), for the purposes of understanding more about the older adults projects we have used and adopted the Maskell Framework from 'The Journey to Agile Manufacturing'.[ii] This framework suggests that agility is a journey through a number of phases, each building on the other.

Foundations

Getting started is about laying down the cornerstones, laying the foundations on which you can build your improvement work. Key factors here are ensuring individuals within teams and teams within organisations have common goals that provide purpose and meaning to their work. The ability to work in teams is essential, as are good communication structures and processes.

Individuals need the basic competencies to carry out their roles and where appropriate, information systems need to support the delivery of care. Structures should be in place to facilitate listening and responding to users and their carers.

Getting cheaper

Once the foundations are in place it is possible to start by reducing the costly activities and concerns. For example, reducing errors, reducing wasteful duplicate handovers and information, reducing the backlog of work, and, where appropriate, reducing costs. It's worth noting, however, that in a complex whole systems environment, improvements made by one agency may result in savings and efficiencies to another.

Getting better

The system is becoming more optimal and now is the time to pay attention to the deeper quality issues. How are the relationships amongst different teams and organisations focused around the needs of the older adult and their pathway of care? How are people within the team and staff in the local community empowered to implement improvements? How have measurements and other quality improvement techniques been used to improve care?

Getting faster

Speeding the processes up can happen in many ways. Synchronising processes helps, as do quick handovers and reducing waiting times. To be successful in this phase, staff need to demonstrate how they are becoming more multi-skilled, working in new areas and in new ways. This is also a phase where performance management becomes part of the system. Success in this phase leads to more satisfactory outcomes for older people and greater efficiency within the system.

Becoming agile

Following all the improvement work, the agile teams, groups and organisations will also maintain an ability to change to meet new demands, and will have accounting and control systems that enable rather than inhibit this. This flexibility will depend on leveraging knowledge and the capability of people within the system.

As you will see from the case studies, this journey is not a linear one. Improvement teams, working with and within their local communities have implemented improvements in ways that best suited their context and the readiness to change by those with whom they were working. Their stories provide evidence of the struggle for excellence, of the need to react to opportunities and the ongoing nature of their work. The case studies outlined below are, as is all continuous improvement work, work in progress.

Case studies

1. Improving the flow of discharge information from hospital to GP

Team Name: Brent Older People's Service
Development Team

Project Manager: Ruth Adam

Key objectives for the project
- To reduce the time taken for discharge information to reach the GP from 9 to 3 days
- To improve the quality of information the GP receives
- For patients to experience a smoother transition from acute to primary care
- To maximise the use of administration time.

Context
Willesden Community Hospital provides a range of rehabilitation and intermediate care facilities. It has 72 in-patient beds, 60 of which are for older people. Patients discharged home from this facility tend to require high level input from community health and social care services.

Establishing foundations
The delay in discharge information reaching the GP was highlighted via a storyboard that mapped an elderly patient's journey through health and social care services in Brent. Both the personal experience of the patient and carer were reflected, as well as pathways of care.

Staff involved in the discharge process were brought together, shown the storyboard and asked to consider the problems and how they might be addressed. This whole systems view helped staff to appreciate the effect of their actions on each other's workload and to focus on improvements for the patient.

The multidisciplinary team mapped out the process from preparing the discharge summary through to the GP responding to it. Problem areas were highlighted and potential solutions agreed.

Getting cheaper

Process redesign involved several key areas that helped reduce waste, costs and mistakes:

- Obtaining a list of fax numbers for all Brent GPs so that the summary could be faxed to the GP prior to posting
- Training ward staff to understanding the importance of completing the summary correctly and agreeing where it would be filed
- Ensuring that pilot practices had systems to bring the discharge to the GP's attention.

The updated process was tested for two weeks and each discharge audited.

Getting better

The team reviewed the results of the audit and identified further areas for improvement, particularly in completing the summary correctly. With management support, a model form was placed on each ward in the discharge tray.

The process was tested and audited for a further two weeks. Sustaining the team's enthusiasm and ensuring continuous improvement involved:

- Use of small scale 'manageable' PDSAs with regular review and feedback
- Management's recognition of the solutions and improvements provided by frontline staff and willingness to implement
- Improved communication outside immediate department
- Simple, continuous measurements, enabling staff to see that today's system needs to be flexible to accommodate tomorrow's changes.

Getting faster

Whilst auditing for sustainability, the delay suddenly increased to 11 days! The key person (admin) who faxed the information had gone on leave. Consequently, two nurses were trained in the discharge process. They faxed the summary to the GP for one week. Finding it did not add significantly to their workload, their suggestion that all nurses could fax the information at the time of discharge to GPs in Brent was tested and implemented.

The administrator who spent many hours chasing lost forms and walking to and from the post room has more time to update the hospital database. GPs receive discharge summaries within 24 hours of discharge (see Figure 9). Patients experience fewer problems with continuing the correct medication on discharge and receiving timely support from their GP and other services.

Becoming agile

Willesden Hospital is now developing a system for planning interdisciplinary patient-focused outcomes of care, involving all departments. By bringing staff together and focusing on the patient experience, barriers are breaking down. It is essential that all staff, including management, are introduced to and understand the value of the collaborative methodology and equipped with the skills to make change manageable and to enable it to co-evolve with new policies, changes of team members and other planned and unexpected events in the future.

Having succeeded in reducing delays in discharge information, a 'can do' environment is developing. People are more open to trying new ways of working. The nature of small scale testing has lent itself well to flexible systems and ongoing review.

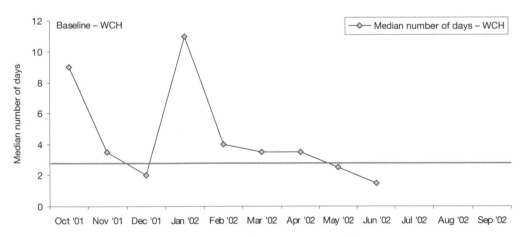

Figure 9: M4(2) – delay in discharge information reaching the GP

2. Development of multidisciplinary community referral form

Team name: Haringey Case Management
                            Collaborative

Project Manager: Alan Beaton

Key objectives for the project
- Map services provided to all users admitted to the project
- Identify gaps and duplication in service provision
- Identify communication difficulties either between services or between services and the user
- Provide focused management and co-ordination of services to achieve the user's personal goals.

Context

In developing the case management process in Haringey, opportunities for the better co-ordination of services to older people were sought. Process mapping was a useful tool for this and brought together a number of disciplines from Community Services and other agencies in the health care environment.

Establishing foundations

This process of mapping the user's journey through the system caused the organisations to start talking together at an operational level. This helped them understand how each other worked and what their priorities and constraints were.

Speedy and effective referrals were recognised as a common goal. The multiplicity of referral forms in use was seen as inefficient and detrimental to a streamlined service. This provided the impetus to make things better and led to the joint development of a multi-purpose referral form.

Getting cheaper

The resulting Multidisciplinary Community Referral Form reduced the need to duplicate information for each referral, cutting out the risk of error. Time was saved further by the inclusion on the form of all the relevant addresses for referral.

The process has been made less onerous, saving the time of the person making the referral and reducing their backlog of work. By relieving this pressure, more thoughtful and better quality referrals are likely to be made, rather than the most expedient.

Getting better

The protocol for use of the form allowed for any health professional to make the referral. The only proviso was that the GP was
informed of and in agreement with the referral. This empowered
the individual practitioner, whilst engendering improved communications and joint working across agencies in the care process.

Getting faster

Quality of care has been further improved by using the referral
form as a trigger for the older person to undergo a period of case
management. Where two or more referrals are made, the case
manager acts as a single point of contact and uses a pro-active
approach to co-ordinate the delivery of care.

Becoming agile

The foundations are being laid for transition to the Single
Assessment Process by this sharing of the referral information.
The form will also lend itself to the development of electronic
records and is being used for the adult population as a whole.

The testing of the form has started with six GP practices. The
rollout will continue as evaluation confirms that improvements to
the delivery of services are being made and that these are sustainable. The work will develop over time to involve other care agencies such as the Intermediate Care team, streamlining referrals in
that environment. Services currently involved in the pilot are all
from the health care sector with capacity for possible rollout to the
social care and independent sectors.

3. Case management in Chiswick

Team name:	Hounslow Older People's Service Development Project
Project Manager:	Keith Strahan

Key objectives for the project
- To ensure that vulnerable older people receive timely, propor-
  tionate, needs led, multi-disciplinary/multi-agency assessment
  as part of the Single Assessment Process
- To improve the co-ordination and integration of the older person's care
- To work in partnership with older people and their carers so
  that they are well informed, actively involved in and have ownership of, their plan of care.

Context

The case management of a complex, high resource user and his carer provided some powerful lessons in the benefits of multi-agency working. Mr T had been living in a nursing home on a privately funded placement for six months, because his wife was no longer able to manage him at home. He was referred to the Primary Care Social Worker (PCSW) for assistance in finding a cheaper nursing home. Initial assessment revealed that Mr T was motivated to return home and this was confirmed by the Primary Care Occupational Therapist (PCOT).

The PCOT became the care co-ordinator, ensuring that a period of six weeks of intensive rehabilitation at an intermediate care centre was followed by the provision of appropriate equipment in the home. The PCSW meanwhile supported Mrs T in preparation for the return of her disabled husband and arranged for an appropriate package of care to help them both. The care co-ordinator role then passed back to the PCSW to assure continuity in the provision of services.

Establishing foundations

A successful development in Hounslow was the attachment of a Primary Care Social Worker to the primary care health team in Chiswick. This proved to be the cornerstone of multi-agency working in the primary care context as it involved collaborative working to achieve positive outcomes for older people. The model is now being spread to the rest of Hounslow.

The flexibility and creativity of the PCSW fostered a willingness to step outside the usual boundaries and helped to produce a local network of agencies committed to working together in the interests of older people.

Getting cheaper

This methodology produced good outcomes, not just for the older person and his carer. Communications were streamlined as the PCSW ensured that all relevant information followed the couple along their journey. This reduced the margin for error and saved practitioners' time.

The care co-ordinator role applied rigour to the process, which meant, with an extremely motivated Mr T, that the care package actually reduced from a long-term nursing place to one hour a day Home Care, resulting in significant cost savings and freeing a nursing home bed.

Getting better

Designating a care co-ordinator at an early stage had an empowering effect, giving the PCOT, and latterly the PCSW, the responsibility to devise, control and integrate the plan of care. It was not a single professional dealing with all the issues in isolation. It was a unified assessment with each professional assisting each other throughout the process.

Getting faster

This case has been used locally as a storyboard to highlight to professionals the importance of:

• joint work between health and social services
• clarification and respect of each other's roles and skills
• sharing information throughout the process.
• Listening to users and their carers and building on their motivation

Becoming agile

As a result of the powerful lessons learnt from this case, a pilot has been developed at the intermediate care centre that will further develop a model of good practice on single assessment and co-ordinated and integrated care.

A major change in procedure has already been agreed in that the Physiotherapist and Occupational Therapist based at the unit can be designated as care co-ordinators. Flexibility in the system is reinforced by their willingness to respond to direct referrals from health and social care professionals (previously only social services departments could refer).

Person-centred care will be achieved, because the older person has that all important, constant 'link' before, during and immediately after leaving the intermediate care centre.

Conclusion

Agility as a concept and philosophy is not only contested but also is in its infancy in the health care sector in the UK. The examples in these case studies show how the concepts can be used to assess progress in improvement work. Although this work is primarily project based, it does demonstrate the usefulness of agility as a framework to guide ambition and sustainability in improvement projects.

9 | Developing agile primary care organisations: using network principles as the basis for organisational design

Maxine Conner, Helen Smith

Introduction

The internal and external operating environment of the primary care organisation requires an organisational design that facilitates the creation of a system that harnesses the talents of the staff who work in a geographical distributed manner. This requires thought and effort, particularly if it is to be agile.

This chapter discusses how the concept of agility can relate to primary care organisations and focuses upon the issue of *connecting* as a means of being agile. Using the ideas of network both as an organisational form and as an approach to organisation design, we consider the issues that face the primary care organisation. This chapter explores the design features of both traditional and networked organisations, providing a comparison with particular emphasis upon the critical issue of responsiveness.

The primary care context

The term 'primary care' is usually defined as the first point of contact with health care services for patients. While this may be true of many patient consultations, the term belies the complexity of what is actually on offer. A huge range of services are provided under this umbrella which include emergency care, treating minor injuries, health promotion, continuing care of elderly patients and those with chronic illnesses, palliative care of those near to death, as well as dental, ophthalmic and pharmaceutical provision. One in four general practitioner (GP) consultations are with people who have mental health problems.[i]

[i] Department of Health, The NHS Plan: A plan for investment: A plan for reform, London HMSO, 2001 (July).

ii The future of UK's family doctors: new contract: www.bma.org.uk/ap.nsf/Content/_Hub+GPC+contract
iii Department of Health, *Shifting the Balance of Power within the NHS – Securing Delivery*, London, HMSO, 2001 (July).

Most staff in more formal primary care settings, such as GP practices, work increasingly in teams, although many community pharmacists, optometrists and, to a lesser extent, dental practitioners continue to work single-handedly and remain relatively isolated from the wider NHS organisation. A broader view of primary care provision could include a long list of less formal agencies and organisations such as family support, alternative therapists, counsellors and many more.

General medical practices have to varying degrees embraced a wide range of government initiatives over the last ten years. The introduction of payments for some individual episodes of care, health promotion targets, fundholding, total purchasing, Personal Medical Services, out-of-hours co-operatives and Specialist GPs have left a legacy of uneven and inequitable provision often accompanied by professional staff who feel a loss of control and who are weary of constant change. A society in which people have become increasingly demanding and litigious and continued government focus on secondary care has contributed to the current challenges.

Many areas of the UK face significant difficulties in recruiting GPs; in some places NHS dentists are simply no longer available. Primary care nevertheless continues to make a valued contribution to health care – patient satisfaction remains very high – both in its own right and as 'gatekeeper' to secondary or hospital care. A revised, more flexible practice-based contract for GPs,[ii] more focused on quality and outcomes is currently under discussion. If adopted, the new contract should help recruitment and retention issues but may result in even greater inequities in provision. These will need to be addressed by primary care organisations.

Primary care organisations

Onto this scene in 2001 arrived 'Primary Care Trusts (PCTs)'. Based as far as possible on natural communities of between 100,000 and 300,000 people, PCTs are charged with[iii]

- Improving the health of the community – a public health role
- Securing the provision of services – a provider and commissioner role
- Integrating health and social care – a modernising role to secure integrated services focused on the needs of patients and users.

To fulfil these roles the new primary care organisations need to work with a vast range of stakeholders …

> 'PCTs will have a clear lead in developing local services and will be able to tailor services to local needs. If this is to be achieved successfully PCTs will need to fully engage their front line staff and local communities and partners in their plans for improving health and health services. The opportunity for PCTs as primarily local organisations to engage and empower **local** communities, patients and frontline staff should bring improvements in local services' (iii).

With wide variations in geography, demography, numbers of staff employed and services provided, some organisations manage a very limited range of community services while others include mental health, community hospitals, rehabilitation and community dental services. Many of these transforming organisations face an immediate and hugely challenging agenda.

They need to acquire or develop new skills in leading change with diverse staff groups; commissioning integrated pathways of care; health surveillance, monitoring and analysis; governance; and genuine public involvement. General practices need to be supported to become more accessible, to audit care, to undertake continuing professional development, to introduce appraisal and to be revalidated. Government targets set out in the NHS plan, National Service Frameworks and other supporting papers must be met within currently very limited resources. The old support networks, Health Authorities and Regional Offices have gone, to be replaced by new Strategic Health Authorities, themselves struggling to come to terms with new and demanding requirements.

To succeed, primary care organisations need to be able to learn quickly. They have to provide fast and flexible services that are able to respond to a myriad of demands within an ever-changing environment. They need to modernise the services for which they are responsible and encourage their stakeholders to be involved in every part of their business.

Designing for agility

Goldman[iv] suggests that agility is …

> 'the capability to co-ordinate quickly and efficiently all of the physically and organisationally distributed resources required to create, produce, deliver and support a constantly changing mix of goods and services …'

[iv] Goldman SL, Graham CB, *Agility in Health Care: Strategies for Mastering Turbulent Markets*, San Francisco, Jossey Bass, 1999.

v Morden T, Principles of Management, London, McGraw-Hill, 1996.
vi Ashkenas R, Ulrich D, Jick T, Kerr S, *The Boundaryless Organisation:Breaking the Chains of Organisational Structure*, San Francisco, Jossey Bass, 1995.
vii Pedler M, Issues in health development: networked organisations – an overview, NHS Development Agency: www.had-online.org.uk, 2001.

To deliver agility within primary care, the organisation must be designed with this goal in sight. The array of both function and people within primary care does not lend itself to the traditional bureaucratic approach to organisational design, developed during the industrial revolution with its emphasis upon control and linearity.[v] The Taylorist principles, which underpin the bureaucratic style, are built upon a traditional mindset, which includes ideas such as:

- People have narrow skills, need to be highly specialised and are easy to replace
- The work has primacy and people must fit around the work
- Staff are cogs in the work machine
- Everything in a work environment can be specified and broken down into simple parts
- The building block for organisational design is one person one task
- High performance will be delivered by supervision and creating competition.

In contrast to this approach, which puts work at the centre and views people as a disposable commodity, networks are designed to be fast and flexible with features synonymous with agility[vi] as described within the chapters of this book. Features, which make networks agile, critically depend upon the connections made between groups and individuals within the system. Pedler[vii] suggests that networks have features that include:

- The linkage of people with common goals
- Values of reciprocity, sharing and mutual interest as core values
- Status and authority that are based upon relationships, knowledge, utility and innovation.

Network design begins from a different base from the traditional bureaucratic principles. This is fundamental to the delivery of speed as a core competency within the organisation. To develop agility and responsiveness two key elements need to be considered: the external operating environment and the educational base of primary care staff. These two features require a different organisational design from that of the traditional hierarchy.

The issue of geography

Primary care staff, although working in teams, do not work in one physical location, they are seldom co-located. They are geographically dispersed. Experience suggests that such staff have a strong sense of identity both with their home team (their practice or functional team) and also their distinct profession. If the essence of agility is to adapt the business to deliver the services needed by the user, then primary care staff need to adapt care delivery, customising and building individual packages of care within varied care settings. As they go about their day-to-day work the team members need to be able to connect rapidly and easily to all parts of the PCT. The issue of connecting people and issues together has far greater significance within this operating environment than in a traditionally hierarchy.

The nature of the workforce

The workforce issues in primary care is complex. Core NHS staff work alongside independent contractors who directly employ their own sub contractors (e.g. practice managers, physiotherapists, counsellors and practise nursing staff), all working to provide care to the patient and commission health services. Our professional staff are highly skilled and educated, and highly trained and committed support staff support work with them. The NHS employs the largest number of graduates in Europe. This demands a change in the way we design the organisation in which primary care staff operate, as the bureaucratic principles around which most organisations are created are not designed to harness the talents of such a group of people.

The organisation design of a PCT must seek to connect and develop the innate ability of the workforce. Making the system agile means enabling the people to work faster and more smoothly. The key to this lies in listening. Staff usually know how to speed up responsiveness; it is the system which prevents them from doing so. The principles identified by Pedler[vii] focus upon the vital element of linkages which need to be a central part of the organisation design within a PCT. Building the linkages delivers a critical element of agility – a connectivity framework. The connectivity needed within PCTs is radically different from building a framework for connecting within a hierarchy.

Networks and their application to primary care

Working with PCTs, it has been possible to explore the opportunities offered by network design principles. Lipnack and Stamps[viii] define networks as ...

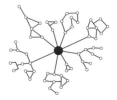

Figure 10

> 'A lumpy organisation of people who deliver a common goal or series of objectives, they are not flat, but multi dimensional, consist of many layers.'

Lumpiness describes the reality of organisational life. People are not just professionals; they are team members in numerous teams.

Consider a woman who is a health visitor in a general practice, who is a team leader for child protection. It is obvious she is part of the practice team, the health visiting team, the child protection team; she has multiple membership. A formal organisational chart will determine where she sits. It is however her own mental model of her work which will determine where she belongs. Her associations and connections determine her success and effectiveness, organisational policies and procedures will guide her practice, but it is her unique understanding, gained through multiple membership that will ensure she is an agile practitioner.

If this is common sense then why is it not common practice? Frequently we experience a managerial mindset within primary care that is based upon traditional bureaucratic principles of *one person – one task*, which marginalises staff from their reality of multiple membership and hinders the effectiveness of the natural connectivity framework within the organisation.

The reality is staff will, if allowed to do so, connect with whom they need to. Being able to do so ensures that decisions are fast and customised solutions can be offered to patients; agility in action?

Within the traditional organisation design, queries and requests for decisions go up and down seeking authorisation at the 'right' level, slowing down the process. The interactions in a network organisation are based upon trust and the application of the education and experience base of the staff. It makes redundant the notion of direct supervision and hierarchical authority based upon position. According to Kiesler and Spoull[ix] ...

> 'In a hierarchy, power is based upon position; in a geographically dispersed organisation it is based upon competency, knowledge and who you connect and collaborate with.'

[viii] Lipnack J, Stamps J, *Virtual Teams*, New York, John Wiley, 2000.
[ix] Kiesler S, Spoull L, 'Reducing social context clues: electronic mail in organisational communication' in: *Connections New Ways of Working in the Networked Organisation*, Cambridge, MIT Press, 1986

The parts of a network

The parts of a network are called nodes. Each node needs to perform its work so that overall the network delivers its goals. Within primary care the practices and the headquarters are nodes. Consider again the idea of 'lumpiness'. PCTs also have health visiting nodes, nodes full of dentists, nodes with public health specialists in them and many others. This is all a matter of how you view the organisation. The traditional mindset requires one to think of the organisation in one dimension, a managerial one, as described by the traditional organisational chart.

However, the design features of a network are based upon multiple membership, providing a multidimensional organisation. Three dimensions appear to exist. You can view the organisation as a series of:

1. Geographical practice based (nodes) groups
2. Professional/functional (nodes) groups
3. Task-based (nodes) groups.

Each grouping can be considered to be a node. All the nodes are valid and represent the reality of primary care. Staff work in many nodes and the connectivity framework must build upon this reality. Understanding the critical work of each node is vital to the development of a cohesive, *response able* organisation. No one node is more important than another, and all are needed to deliver the business of the organisation.

However each node is likely to be different as they may have different functions to perform and perform them in different ways. However they will have some common functions. The key issue here is about clarity of purpose within the nodes.

Consider the following examples:

The GP practice as a node

Within primary care the practices are nodes, each one with services to provide. Each practice may do so in a different way, a way that suits its particular patient populations and locality. From a managerial perspective there needs to be clarity of WHAT each node should contribute to deliver the overall goals. The process of 'how' is important and should be worked out locally within the nodes, as the staff within the practice (node) understand the local context best of all.

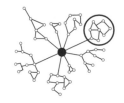

Figure 11

Primary care management team as a node

Within a primary care organisation the managerial team are also a node. The managerial node is no more or less important than the practice nodes, it just has a different function.

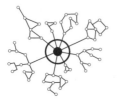

Figure 12

In the same way that the practice nodes must work out their purpose, the purpose and function of the management node is part of the critical design element. The critical element for any managerial team within a network is the issue of what they focus upon, and the level of hierarchy it takes to make a decision. Too many levels of hierarchy result in slow responses.

In an agile organisation, communication and connectivity is open and fluid, with people talking to whom they need to, in order to get the job done or the problem resolved. Decisions must be made at the most appropriate point in the organisation to achieve a fast 'customer' responses. Deferring decisions to the PCT management team, should only be done where it makes sense to do so, if speed is to be a feature within primary care.

A profession task group as a node

In this example the lines connect some district nurses within the PCT. They have geographically distributed bases, but come together as a professional node.

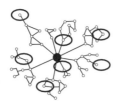

Figure 13

Conclusion

x Kostner J, *Virtual Leadership*, London, Warner Business Books, 1996.

In agile organisations a connectivity framework exists which enables the different nodes to function effectively together. Kostner[x] suggests that distance is the enemy of staff and managers within a geographically distributed organisation. Attention to the concept of connectivity is needed to overcome this issue. Building and maintaining commitment to the purpose of the organisation requires managers to build the connectivity framework, with common processes, which can be locally adapted to the external environment and which deliver the overall business of the PCT. Agile organisations react fast to change but use a range of approaches, which ensure rapid communication not hindered by distance.

Kanter[xi] sums up the challenge of designing an agile primary care organisation when she states ...

> 'It requires more agile, limber management that pursues opportunity without being bogged down by cumbersome structures or weighty procedures that impede action.'

The question is can our primary care organisations rise to the challenge?

[xi] Kanter RM, *When Giants Learn to Dance*, London, International Thomson Business Press, 1998.

10 | Performance managing agile organisations

Barry Tennison, David J. Yarrow

Defining some terms

This chapter sets out to explore performance management in agile organisations. Before we go any further, it would be helpful to define some terms.

Let's start with 'performance'. Unsurprisingly, the NHS Plan places emphasis on performance:

'The NHS is a 1940s system operating in a 21st century world. It has … a lack of national standards … [and] … a lack of clear incentives and levers to improve performance.'[i]

What exactly do we mean by '*performance*'? A dictionary definition is 'something that is carried out or accomplished'.[ii] If the organisation achieves its goals, then it has performed. This sounds simple enough, but in practice things are a little more complex (or, perhaps, we *make things* more complex, when we should really be clinging on to the simplicity?). The dictionary also offers an alternative definition: 'a presentation of an artistic work to an audience, for example a play or piece of music'.[iii] This could easily be dismissed as a different meaning of the same word, but perhaps we should ponder for a moment which of these definitions is most relevant to much of the measurement and 'performance management' that goes on from day to day in real organisations.

Performance management of staff is an approach to linking an individual's objectives, performance and development to the strategic aims of the organisation.[iv,v] While it has come to prominence in recent years, its roots can be traced to 'scientific management' as described by Taylor[vi] in the early 20th century, and it draws heavily upon the 'management by objectives' principles[vii] and more recent approaches including the widespread implementation of appraisal schemes and of the Investors in People standard,[viii] and the 'balanced scorecard'[ix] approach to performance measurement.

[i] Department of Health, *The NHS Plan: a Plan for Investment: a Plan for Reform. A Summary*, HMSO, London, 2000 (July), p. 2.

[ii] *Encarta World English Dictionary*, Microsoft Corporation, 1999.

[iii] Ibid.

[iv] goodpractice.net, *The Importance of Performance Management – an Overview*, www.goodpractice.net, 24th March 2002.

[v] Armstrong M, Baron A, *Performance Management: The New Realities*, Institute of Personnel and Development, London, 1998.

[vi] Taylor FW, 'Shop Management' in *Scientific Management*, Harper & Row: USA, 1964 (original article written in 1911)

[vii] Drucker PF, *Management: Tasks, Responsibilities, Practices*, Heinemann, London, 1974.

[viii] Investors in People, *Investors in People: The context*, www.iipuk.co.uk/investorsinpeople/thestandard/, 18th October 2002.

[ix] Kaplan R, Norton D, 'Balanced Scorecard: measures that drive performance', *Harvard Business Review*, January–February 1992.

x goodpractice.net,
Performance management – Effective Management Practice – Good Practice: AA Insurance, www.goodpractice.net, 24th March 2002

xi goodpractice.net,
Performance management – Effective management practice – Good Practice: Volkswagen, www.goodpractice.net, 24th March 2002

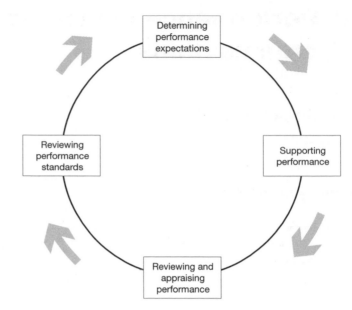

Figure 14: The performance management cycle

Adapted from Torrington D and Hall L, *Personnel Management: Human Resource Management in Action*, Prentice Hall, 1995

Performance managing staff has been credited as an important component in the success of some progressive organisations,[x,xi] helping them to effect changes and improve outcomes. Described as a cyclical process, it focuses attention upon the individual's competencies and development, in order to ensure that they are capable of playing their part in the overall performance of the organisation.

Performance management of organisations usually occurs in a system of organisations with different roles. For example in markets or pseudo-markets, there are often organisations charged with

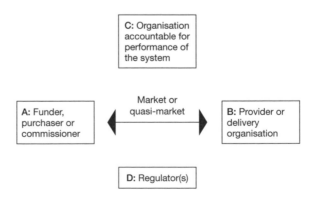

Figure 15: Organisational systems

Table 5: Health care organisations and roles

	A: Funder	B: Deliverer	C: Accountable	D: Regulator
NHS in 1990s	Health authorities	NHS trusts	Department of Health and Regional Offices	Department of Health and Regional Offices
NHS in 2000s	Primary care trusts, plus specialist commissioners	NHS trusts and primary care trusts	Department of Health through DHSCs and Strategic health authorities	Commission for Health Improvement (CHI), National Patient Safety Agency (NPSA) etc
Financial services market	Purchasers and investors, individual and institutional	Providers of financial services	Stakeholders, shareholders and customers	Financial Services Agency (FSA)
'Best Value' in local authority services	Local people through local authorities (some via central taxation)	In house services and outsourcing providers	Local and central government	Audit Commission
Education (England)	Central government	Schools and colleges	Central government	Office for Standards In Education (OFSTED)

regulating or overseeing the system, in particular seeing that market rules are obeyed. There may also be organisations (or parts of the system) that have the role of developing or managing the performance of other parts of the system. A general scheme is given in Figure 15.

Some examples of systems and the organisations with different roles are given in Table 5.

Performance management within organisations: theory into practice

At first sight, the logic of performance management of individuals is difficult to fault. Undoubtedly, a well-implemented approach embodying these principles would be an asset to an organization which seeks to set ambitious goals and then to achieve them, mobilising its entire workforce to good effect in order to do so. However, several key questions need to be answered:

- Is performance management invariably 'well-implemented'? What are the pitfalls? Is there a danger that good intentions

[xii] Neely A, *Measuring Business Performance – Why, What and How*, Profile Books Ltd, London, 1998, p. 1

[xiii] Ibid., p. 3

translate to a counter-productive regime with sub-optimisation as its net effect?

- Does performance management tend to act as an enabler of change (and agility), or as an inhibitor?

Like so many of the tools and approaches that are deployed in organisations, performance management is as good as the skills of the people deploying it and the way they set about the task. Senior management's role is crucial in determining if the commitment to the approach is genuine, sustained, properly resourced and regularly reinforced. Are the leaders prepared to take their own medicine, and be seen to be doing so? So too are the skills and attitudes of those who review performance, at all levels, and the basis on which judgements are made and feedback provided. And decisions regarding the nature of measurement and communication, at the macro and micro levels, will make or break performance management's credibility and effects.

Andy Neely in his book 'Measuring Business Performance – why, what and how' asks why so many people are so interested in business performance measurement today:

'The main theme of the book is that the traditional view of measurement as a means of control is naïve. As soon as performance measures are used as a means of control, the people being measured begin to manage the measures rather than the performance.'[xii]

He identifies three roles of measurement – comply, check and challenge – which he sees as:

'...significantly different from and much richer than the traditional view of measurement as a means of control. They are not based on the assumption that the behaviour of people can be controlled through measurement. They are founded on the assumptions that measurement is a tool to be used by people to enhance business performance and that there are distinct dimensions of business performance, which need to be measured and managed in different ways.'[xiii]

Table 6 illustrates multiple reasons for measuring ('the four CPs').

Within any individual organisation, the emphases that are embodied in the approach to performance measurement and management will determine whether the regime is one that supports and enables improving performance, flexibility and agility, or one that imposes constraints and acts as a strait-jacket. Is the emphasis on setting direction, communicating position, supporting understanding and learning and enabling change? Or is it on control, compliance, standardisation and conformity? As a

Table 6

Why measure?

CP1: check position
- Measures as a means of establishing position
- Measures as a means of comparing position (benchmarking)
- Measures to monitor progress

CP2: communicate position
- Measures as a means of communicating performance
- Measuring because you have to: communicating with the regulator

CP3: confirm priorities
- Measures to manage
- Measures as a means of management and cost control
- Measures to make clear
- Measures as a means of focusing investment

CP4: compel progress
- Measures as a means of motivation
- Measures as a means of communicating priorities
- Measures as a basis for reward

Source: Neely A, *Measuring Business Performance – Why, What and How*, Profile Books Ltd., London, 1998, p. 89.

customer-facing employee in this organisation, is performance management something that is done *for me*, to help me to better serve the unique ever-evolving needs of our individual clients?; or something that is done *to me*, as a means of controlling me, checking my conformance to the rules, keeping me 'in line' with others' pre-determined policies and plans?

Performance management of organisations: performance indicators

When managing the performance of organisations within a system (like a market or quasi-market), the 'four CPs' table again gives compelling reasons why measurement is a key issue. This is why *performance indicators* (PIs) have become a basic tool of performance management. For many organisations, as noted at the beginning of this chapter, performance is a complicated matter. It can include:

- for a commercial organisation, satisfying shareholders as well as employees, and fulfilling obligations to society

xiv Freeman T, Using performance indicators to improve health care quality in the public sector: a review of the literature. *Health Services Management Research* 15: 126–137, 2002.

- for a voluntary organisation, satisfying its clients as well as its funders
- for a public sector organisation, satisfying local or central government (who hold legislative and purse strings as well as expressing collective will) while serving its customers (who may be alienated from government aims)
- for a health care provider, satisfying patient needs, professional objectives (including 'best possible care' as well as aspirations for status and employment benefits), public pressures and government aims.

Performance indicators for the NHS have been refined over a number of years (see http://www.doh.gov.uk/nhsperformanceindicators). They are currently based on a 'performance assessment framework' with six dimensions (for funders/commissioners of care):

1. Health improvement
2. Fair access
3. Effective delivery of appropriate care
4. Efficiency
5. Patient/carer experience
6. Health outcomes of NHS care

which (despite the obscuring effects of shorthand technical terms) reveal the multiple pressures and objectives. There is a similar performance assessment framework for NHS trusts and another for personal social services.

The account of the performance of NHS health authorities in England, published in February 2002, contains, for each of the ninety or so health authorities, the values of about fifty performance indicators. This is a formidable amount of data, whether for the public or for those who are trying to improve performance.

There is a considerable literature on using performance indicators to improve health care quality.xiv Freeman makes the distinction between the uses of performance indicators as:

- summative mechanisms for external accountability and verification; and/or
- formative mechanisms for internal quality improvement.

There is a venerable tradition of different views being taken on the same performance indicators. For sophisticated regulators and performance managers, they are seen as 'simply' indicators of where there might be relative or absolute problems; adverse values imply the need for further investigation, or attention to a particular area. Those whose performance is being measured are more likely to see them as quantities that have to be got 'right' to free them from undesired interference. This often leads to the reactions of: trying to show the value is incorrect; denigrating the usefulness of the indicator; or in some cases manipulating data or data systems to ensure favourable figures.

Freeman, adapting Smith,[xv] expands this to a table of unintended consequences of public sector performance indicator systems:

[xv] Smith P, The unintended consequences of publishing performance data in the public sector. *International Journal of Public Administration* 18(2): 277–310, 1995.

Tunnel vision	Emphasis on phenomena quantified in the measurement scheme
Sub-optimisation	Pursuit of narrow local objectives, rather than those of the whole organisation or system
Myopia	Pursuit of short term targets
Measure fixation	Pursuit of strategies enhancing the measure rather than the associated objective
Misrepresentation	Deliberate manipulation of data
Misinterpretation	Drawing misleading inferences from raw performance data
Gaming	Deliberate manipulation of behaviour to secure strategic advantage
Ossification	Organisational paralysis due to rigid performance evaluation.

If we are to encourage agility, and use measurement to do so, how can we avoid these pitfalls and develop agility as part of developing performance?

Performance management or performance development?

It is all too easy for performance management to be seen simply as 'checking up'. At its worst, it identifies departures from desired performance based on simplistic measures, and then dispenses punishment. In some systems (for example, training a conditioned reflex or a neural network) this may be appropriate; but for complex human systems, experience teaches that it is seldom a way to improve performance, especially when the actual outcomes desired are multidimensional and complexly interrelated. And when the punishment involves removal of resources (human, financial or other), why should improvement be expected, unless the removed factors are known to be holding back improvement?

It can be fruitful to deliberately replace the term 'performance management' by 'performance development'. This acknowledges the idea that those who are trying to improve a system need both

- to encourage improvement through positive enabling steps; and
- to enhance the capacity and capability of organisations (and individuals) to improve.

For example, the too frequent response to an adverse performance indicator value (especially one of long standing) is a conversation between a defensive (non-) performer and an exasperated performance manager. It is not necessarily easy to turn this into a constructive examination of:

- whether there is a problem (without defensiveness)
- if so, of what nature
- what means might be useful in tackling it
- who is actually going to do what, when.

Some tools that aid this are:

- sympathy and sense of proportion
- specific efforts to gain ownership and commitment, before moving on
- techniques like root cause analysis to dig behind simplistic answers to 'why?' – often involving a range of stakeholders
- systems diagnosis rather than ascriptions to specific individuals or teams
- action planning, usually involving a range of stakeholders
- judicious use of external help and resources
- efforts to think radically and go for radical rather than incremental improvement.

Many of the approaches and techniques being used by the NHS Modernisation Agency are moves in this direction, for example the 'Pursuing Perfection' programme (see http://www.ihi.org/pursuingperfection/ and the results of a Google search on 'pursuing perfection').

Performance management and agility: friends or foes?

Turning again to the dictionary to remind ourselves of the meaning of 'agility':

1. physical nimbleness: a combination of physical speed, suppleness, and skill
2. mental alertness: a combination of mental quickness, alertness, and intelligence'[xvi]

The concept of agility in the organisational sense has developed from a recognition that, although some manufacturing businesses have developed to a point where they may be considered 'lean', this may not be sufficient for them to cope and excel in today's fast-moving environment. Table 7 shows five key principles which are said to characterise lean systems.

Agile manufacturing is a step on from 'lean'. The characteristics of lean production are extended to encompass the following four basic principles:[xvii]

[xvi] *Encarta World English Dictionary*, op. cit.

[xvii] Goldman SL, Agile competitors and virtual organizations: strategies for enriching the customer, Van Nostrand Reinhold, 1994 (cited in Robertson, M and Jones, C, Application of lean production and agile manufacturing concepts in a telecommunications environment, *International Journal of Agile Management Systems*, 1(1), 1999).

Table 7: Five key principles which characterize lean systems

1: Value	Precisely specify value by specific product/service	Redefine the whole product/service through the eyes of the customer
2: Value stream	Identify the value stream for each product/service	This is the entire set of actions required to bring the product/service from its raw materials/initiation to the customer
3: Flow	Make value flow without interruptions	Eliminate departmentalisation and batch processing so that the process can flow, leading to a short lead-time, high quality and low cost
4: Pull	Let the customer pull value from the producer	If lead-times are reduced, then a producer can design, schedule and make/deliver exactly what the customer wants, when (s)he wants it, rather than relying on a demand forecast. In practice, pull is usually achieved using the system known as 'just-in-time' (JIT). JIT is a system whereby an upstream process does not produce parts until requested by a down-stream process.
5: Perfection	Pursue perfection	Do not attempt to be slightly better than your competitors/peers, but rather strive for perfection through the use of continuous improvement

Adapted from: Robertson, M and Jones, C, Application of lean production and agile manufacturing concepts in a telecommunications environment, *International Journal of Agile Management Systems*, 1(1), 1999, pp. 14–16

xviii Dove R, Knowledge management, response ability, and the agile enterprise, *Journal of Knowledge Management*, 3(1), 1999, pp. 18–35

xix Ibid., p. 18.

1. Products are solutions to customers' individual problems.
2. Virtual organisations are formed where products are brought to market in minimum time through internal and external co-operation.
3. Entrepreneurial approaches are adopted so that organisations thrive on change and uncertainty.
4. Knowledge-based organisations are formed which focus on distributed authority supported by information technology.

There is an emphasis here on flexibility, adaptability, responsiveness and change. Distributed authority enables individuals and teams who work directly with the customers to tailor and evolve their products and services to the requirements they are encountering and analysing day-to-day and hour-to-hour.

Like change itself, agility is nothing new.[xviii] It has always been necessary for organisations to be sufficiently agile to adjust and adapt to their changing environment. What is different today is the greater pace of change, which brings into sharp focus an organisation's agility, or lack of it. Whereas previously the organisation might evolve at a relatively comfortable pace, perhaps almost unconsciously, there is now a need to hone the competencies of adaptation, so that they can be deployed faster and better than before. The pressure is on.

The situation could be likened to a competent driver, with years of experience of coping with the demands of urban and motorway driving, being suddenly asked to get behind the wheel of a racing car and compete on a demanding racetrack. The driver finds that he is acutely conscious of every action, every movement, every new piece of information which his senses must process in order to determine an appropriate response. Having progressed during his early learning experiences through the stages of learning to a state of unconscious competence, he now feels that he has suddenly regressed. He is consciously incompetent to deal with the demands of this new environment. To survive, he must consciously focus upon the skills and actions that will enable him to perform, to gain experience, to err and learn, and ultimately to recapture the status of unconscious competence that will enable him to excel at a whole new level.

The key enablers of agility have been identified as *knowledge management* and *change proficiency*, leading to a useful and succinct definition of agility as:

'the ability to manage and apply knowledge effectively.'[xix]

How comfortably, then, will the development of organisational agility co-exist with a framework of performance management? The answer, perhaps predictably, is 'it depends'. If the implementation of performance management is in reality an attempt to control and to ensure conformance to pre-determined and inflexible standards and norms, then there is no doubt that this regime and efforts to develop agile competencies will be in direct conflict. Agility requires a freedom to adapt, to change, to learn, to review, and to adapt again. My performance, in a narrow sense of the word, will almost certainly not be what I thought it would be several months ago. I didn't know then what the requirements were going to be, so how could I possibly predict the performance?

If, on the other hand, the implementation of performance management is at the more 'enlightened' end of the spectrum, then agility may find itself being nurtured in a more conducive environment. Individuals and teams are empowered to sense and respond to the unique and evolving requirements of the patients and service users they encounter, unencumbered by rigid targets or norms that would constrain their ability to design and deliver the required service. Meanwhile, the performance management cycle is applied to good effect at a 'higher level', monitoring and analysing changes and trends in expectations and feedback, managing new knowledge and making it available in a timely and effective manner, and enabling the development of the competencies which underpin agility and performance.

For performance management and agility to work together in harmony, there needs to be an understanding of performance

---

Box 9: Rick Dove offers an illuminating simile

Agile is a word we associate with cats. When we associate a cat as being agile we are observing that it is both physically adept at movement and also mentally adept at choosing useful movement appropriate for the situation. Agile carries with it the elements of timeliness and grace and purpose and benefit as well as nimbleness.

A cat that simply has the ability to move quickly, but moves inappropriately and to no gain might be called reactionary, spastic, or confused, but never agile. Picture a cat on a hot tin roof.

Conversely, a cat that knows what should be done but finds itself unable to move might be called afraid, catatonic, or paralysed, but never agile. Like the cat that's got itself up a tree.

Source: Dove R, Knowledge management, response ability, and the agile enterprise, *Journal of Knowledge Management*, 3(1), 1999, p. 20

which accommodates uncertainty and change, and a willingness to 'manage' in the sense of providing leadership and support rather than an emphasis on commanding and controlling. At the local level, performance is ultimately about fulfilling the requirements of this individual patient, now, albeit that those requirements might be unpredictable in detail and quite different from those of the previous patient or the next one. Local measures and feedback must be supportive to these needs, not counter-productive, constraining and undertaken only to feed a remote, 'central' need rather than to develop useful, timely knowledge.

Today's organisation needs to display the mental and physical agility of the cat, not the panic of the rabbit in the headlights.

11 | Coping with uncommon calamities: building safer systems

David Aron

Introduction

Organisational agility, shorthand for a complex, context-sensitive response-ability, has been proposed as a business strategy for successful mastery of rapidly changing, intensely competitive markets.[i] In addition to being characterised by efficient production/ provision of quality products/services, such organisations possess 'the capability to coordinate quickly and efficiently all of the physically and organisationally distributed resources required to create, produce, deliver, and support a constantly changing mix of goods and services for fickle markets.'[ii] An important characteristic of these markets is their requirement for meeting the unique needs of individual customers – one size does not fit all. Although proposed for profit-driven business, similar principles apply to the non-profit sector in general and health care in particular.

For example, consider the hospital casualty department or emergency room (ER). The service, health care, is provided to all. However, each patient presents with different problems and unique needs. A patient with a minor illness might be treated by a single physician based solely on that physician's examination. A motor vehicle accident victim may require the coordinated efforts of a trauma team of highly specialised individuals plus a wide variety of services from throughout the hospital and beyond (e.g. regional blood bank). Thus, ERs exhibit many of the characteristics of agility such as support for pervasive cooperative relationships across the organisation and with other organisations, and deeply distributed authority with strategically coordinated decentralised decision-making. These and other agility principles can be applied at a broader organisational level in the health care system.

For health care organisations, functioning in today's complex and changing environment, potential calamity lurks at every turn. Such organisations must continually adapt and improve and by

[i] Goldman SL, Graham C (eds) *Agility in Health Care: Strategies for Mastering Turbulent Markets*. Jossey-Bass, 1999.

[ii] Ibid.

iii Perrow C, *Normal Accidents*. New York, Basic Books, 1999.

iv Berniker E, Wolf F, *Managing Complex Technical Systems Working on a Bridge of Uncertainty* http://www.plu.edu/ ~bernike/ManComSys/ Managing%20Complex SystemsIAMOT.doc accessed July 8, 2002.

co-evolving with changing conditions must attend to the importance of defending against failure. Coping with uncommon calamities requires building safer systems.

In this chapter we address the issues of organisational vulnerability and organisational resilience, focusing not on classical crisis management, but rather in what it takes to create (and re-create) such safer systems.

Organisational vulnerability and the inevitability of calamity

The term organisational accident usually refers to calamities that involve loss of life or major societal disruption such as a nuclear power plant accident. Charles Perrow studied the Three Mile Island accident and introduced the concepts of 'normal accidents'.[iii] He theorised that the combination of two factors – *complexity* and *tight coupling* – made accidents inevitable.

Technological systems typically are characterised by numerous interconnections and potential interactions among subsystems, i.e. *complexity*. This complexity ensures that there will be unexpected, unpredictable, and not readily comprehensible interactions between independent failures. *Tight coupling* in which sub-components have prompt and major impacts on each other ensures that the ensuing failures will be propagated. With so many interconnections, several supposedly independent sub-components may fail simultaneously, escalating from small failures to a major calamity or as the adage goes: 'For want of a nail … a kingdom was lost.' Perrow also classified a number of industries based on these two characteristics (see Figure 16).

A different way of thinking about this theory is in terms of one of the fundamental laws of physics, the second law of thermodynamics which states that all systems must move towards increasing entropy or disorder. 'Any system of sufficient complexity and tightness of coupling must, over time, exhibit entropic behavior and uncertainty resulting in its failure. Failure is a certainty and, therefore, recovery and repair must be possible for the system to avoid end state equilibrium. In the case of complex, tightly coupled systems, we simply cannot know enough about them to anticipate all modes of failure and prevent them within the time and resources available.'[iv]

In fact, even efforts to maintain order are doomed to failure; technical or non-technical safety measures may increase the complexity and or tighten the coupling resulting in either more

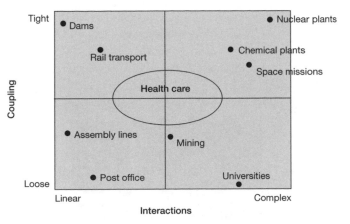

Perrow, 1999

Figure 16: Classification of Industries/Organisations Based on Levels of Coupling and Complexity. Processes in health care may fit in any of the quadrants (modified from www.eng.uwaterloo.ca/~sd142/material/notes/system.ppt after Perrow, 1999 – accessed July 8, 2002).

[v] McNutt R, Abrams R, Aron DC for the Patient Safety Committee. Patient safety efforts should focus on medical errors. *JAMA* 287:1997–2001, 2002.

[vi] Berniker E, Wolf F, ibid.

[vii] Evan WM, Manion M. *Minding the Machines: Preventing Techno-logical Disasters.* Prentice Hall PTR, Upper Saddle River, New Jersey, 2002.

[viii] Reason J, *Managing the Risks of Organizational Accidents.* Aldershot, UK, Ashgate Publishing Ltd, 1997.

unexpected interactions or more rapid propagation of failure or both. For example, computerisation of physician order entry has been proposed as a method to decrease the number of medication errors. However, order entry may lead to other sorts of injury if the system of care in which order entry resides is not clearly organised to maximize the benefits.[v] Computerisation can increase both the tightness of the coupling and complexity resulting in new vulnerabilities. Technology can indeed bite back.

This suggests that basic safety systems will never be sufficient: better run organisations will have fewer discrete errors available for unexpected interactions that can defeat safety systems, but those errors cannot be reduced to zero.[vi] While Perrow emphasises technology, it is important not to neglect the integral part played by individuals.[vii] Technological disasters result from interactions between individuals and technology in the context of organisations and society. Individuals (and organisations) may be involved in accident causation, but they also play a critical part in accident prevention (see below). In fact, sometimes they may have to respond to circumstances and break the 'safety rules' for the sake of safety.

An important conceptual breakthrough in understanding organisational accidents was the differentiation between two types of failure – *active* and *latent*.[viii]

Active failures are often attributed to the actions of visible operators of the system at the human-system interface, e.g. the

ix Pidgeon N, The Limits to Safety? Culture, Politics, Learning and Man-Made Disasters. *Journal of Contingencies and Crises Management* 5(1), March 1997.

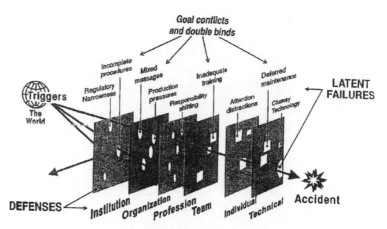

Figure 17: Swiss Cheese Model of Defenses Against Failure (www.vipcs.org/conf2001/vipcs041701.ppt from James Reason, 1991 – accessed July 8, 2002)

nuclear plant control room supervisor or airline pilot. Humans may make the active errors that precipitate the adverse event, but these errors are symptoms of other, deeper system problems – latent failures. These latent failures lie dormant within a technological system and do not in themselves cause an accident or incident. All hazardous technologies possess layers of barriers and safeguards. These defenses take a variety of forms – technological, administrative, educational, and cultural. Ideally, in combination the defensive layers would be impermeable.

However, in reality, there are always weaknesses in the defences. The layers are more like slices of Swiss cheese, containing many holes that are continually opening, shutting, and altering their positions (see Figure 17). Fortunately, because there are multiple layers, the presence of holes in any one 'slice' normally does not cause a bad outcome. If there is a hole in one, another defence will prevent the hazard from causing damage. However, latent errors can build up and the holes in many layers line up to permit a trajectory of accident opportunity-bringing hazards. The complexity of the system may allow the unappreciated build-up of latent failures and the consequent risk of a major system failure. This collective failure of 'intelligence' results both from the underlying complexity of the system and also from the fact that the systems are socio-technical in nature and subject to all the limitations to which human systems are prone.[ix]

Modern health care delivery involves complex socio-technical systems managing a series of complex problems. Although individual components of a system may be simplified, simplification as an overarching strategy to deal with complexity is not possible. The need for specialisation and division of labour has led to the phenomenon of 'structural secrecy' or compartmentalisation of knowledge and information.[x,xi] Moreover, health care delivery takes place in a complex and rapidly changing environment. This environment brings with it new systemic vulnerabilities (and attenuates or eliminates old ones). In addition to this increasing complexity, the drive for greater efficiency in response to economic pressure often involves tighter coupling as redundancy is removed from the system. Complexity and tight coupling present serious risk and even with the best intentions of all concerned, calamities take place.

Organisational resilience and management of the unexpected

Despite the rather depressing prospect of the inevitability of failure, some organisations have managed (with the consciousness that this term should imply) to greatly reduce the frequency or maintain low rates of catastrophic failure. These organisations have been termed 'high reliability organisations' (HROs).[xii] These organisations operate in highly complex and technologically hazardous arenas such as aviation and nuclear power where the potential for catastrophic misadventure is great.

HROs are characterised by the priority given by top management to safety and reliability, decentralised and continually practiced team-based operations, a flattened hierarchy, high levels of redundancy in order to back-up failing technology and people, and a high reliability or safety culture. In a safety-oriented culture, human error is accepted as a fact of life that must be managed rather than an individual moral failing that can be eliminated. There is continual reflection upon practice through monitoring, analysis and feedback systems, which to be effective must be done in a non-punitive manner.

Consequently, cooperation, collaboration and communication are highly valued. Similarly, because there is much to be learned from near misses in which no adverse outcome was experienced, value placed on reporting them; anomalies are goads to reflection. In fact, anomalies must be actively sought out because success is thought to breed complacency. In trying to prepare for emergencies, they are rehearsed. These and other characteristics facilitate both individual and organisational learning that helps to prepare for the unforeseeable.

[x] West E, Organisational sources of safety and danger: sociological contributions to the study of adverse events. *Quality in Health care* 9:120–126, 2000.

[xi] Vaughan D. *The Challenger Launch Decision*. Chicago, University of Chicago Press, 1996.

[xii] Weick KE, Sutcliffe KM. *Managing the Unexpected: Assuring High Performance in an Age of Complexity*. New York, Jossey-Bass, 2001.

A safer system does a better job of detecting the weak signals of an unexpected event in the making and by responding strongly halts the cascading impact early. When this cannot be done, a safer system does a better job at containment. When containment fails, the safer system's resilience permits it to bounce back quickly and focus on restoration of system functioning. All organisations try to accomplish this. The success of HROs, particularly in their higher sensitivity to the weak signals of low level discrepant events has been attributed to their efforts to act mindfully. This mindful approach is a form of continuous sensemaking and well-developed situational awareness. The ability to sense and respond to changing conditions is the essence of agility. Hindsight allows us to see what the warning signs were. It is not easy to detect a signal over the baseline level of random 'noise' in real time. Such low level discrepant events are often explained away as it may be easier from a psychological standpoint to construct non-threatening explanations, a concept referred to as normalisation of deviance. This sensitivity to discrepant events is reflected in a preoccupation with failure in which any lapse is seen as a symptom of an underlying system problem that could escalate into a calamity.

Functional and organisational redundancies contribute to overall system safety. This phenomenon refers to the presence of backup systems, both technical and human. HROs are characterised by high levels of redundancy and go several steps beyond cross-functional training. Overlapping competence is important in ensuring the possibility of individuals monitoring the performance of each other in a meaningful way. Moreover, there are patterns of co-operation that foster interactions among knowledgeable colleagues, i.e. knowledge transfer and a willingness to defer to expertise as opposed to experience, the latter by itself being no guarantee of the former. The safety culture reinforces the willingness to intervene and be intervened upon, regardless of rank. HROs also change their interaction styles depending upon the demands. Under normal circumstances, formal lines of authority are the rule. In a crisis, expertise 'outranks' hierarchy. Resilience also requires the ability to improvise so that the system continues to function. Such improvisation in turn requires a deep knowledge of the technology, the system, one's co-workers, one's self, and other resources.

It is knowledge management in action.

The relationship between *agility* and building safer systems

Agility is the ability to manage and apply knowledge effectively, i.e. the combination of knowledge management plus *response ability*. Designing an agile system means designing sustainable proficiency at change into the very nature of the system.[xiii] The principles of agility provide a conceptual framework for building safer systems.

Change agility is the capacity to effectively respond, anticipate and be generative in relation to a changing environment and to bring a degree of newness to familiar and habitual patterns. It involves not just the speed of response to change in the environment, but also the purposiveness, flexibility, depth/breadth and perceptiveness of the response. Change agility is something that enables the organisation to better serve its wider community needs.[xiv] Some agile system principles include non-hierarchical interaction, distributed control and information, self-organising relationships, flexible capacity, unit redundancy. These principles and others parallel those that facilitate the development and operation of HROs.

For example, in the agile organisation, it is recognised that further change will always be necessary so that proficiency at change is stressed more than any single successful change. The value of management coaching versus management control is reflected in the HROs' practice of deference to expertise, especially in a crisis. The concern for entrepreneurship and improvisation versus working to job descriptions is reflected in the HRO commitment to resilience. The emphasis on learning from outcomes – knowledge creation and management versus mere accumulation of items of knowledge is mirrored in the HRO perspectives of collaborative inquiry and preoccupation with failure. When solutions as opposed to goods and services are more highly regarded, system redesign is easier. Reconfigurability is stressed as contrasted with operational efficiency and workforce adaptability rather than specific skills. This is not to say that a safer system can be built from totally unskilled personnel, but rather that workers who can continually learn new skills will be better able to adjust to the inevitable changing conditions.[xv]

Finally, an HRO will take assistance wherever it can find it. The agile enterprise values relationships with customers as opposed to simple transactions. This facilitates partnering with customers who are in fact part of the system. Patients have a great deal to add to making the health care system safer.

[xiii] Dove R. *Design Principles for Highly Adaptable Business Systems, With Tangible Manufacturing Examples.* www.parshift.com/docs/ RrsPrinciplesMIH.htm accessed July 8, 2002.

[xiv] Binns P. The Change Agile Organisation. www.ie.edu/efmd/ documents/The_Agile _Organisation.ppt accessed April 17, 2002.

[xv] Fraser SW, Greenhalgh T. Complexity science: coping with complexity: educating for capability. *BMJ* 323:799–803, 2001.

Conclusion

All large complex systems have risks and hazards intrinsic to performing their functions. Health care systems operate in complex environments where pressure to improve all dimensions of performance is the norm. These complex internal and external environments are always changing thus increasing the threat of unpredictable events. Organisational resilience has traditionally depended on the extraordinary capacity of humans to bounce back from adversity. Resilient organisations harness that capacity more effectively and link it to its technical assets. Building a safer system requires both ability to adapt to the unexpected and resilience in order to detect the weak signals of an unexpected event in the making, to respond strongly at an early point, to contain failure, and restore system functioning. Enterprises can organise for adaptability and resilience. The principles of agility provide a framework that can facilitate the development of safer systems.

Table 8: Tight vs. loose coupling*

Tight coupling	Loose coupling
Delays in processing not possible	Delays in processing possible
Invariant sequences	Order of sequences can be changed
Only one method to achieve goal	Alternative methods available
Little slack possible in supplies, equipment, personnel	Slack in resources possible
Buffers and redundancies designed-in, deliberate	Buffers and redundancies fortuitously available
Substitutions for supplies, equipment, personnel limited and designed-in	Substitutions fortuitously available

*(www.cis.drexel.edu/faculty/robertson/courses/isys110/Slides/Accidents.ppt after Perrow, 1999 – accessed July 8, 2002)

Table 9. Building a high reliability organization: key factors to assess in the institution, organization, or department*

- Overall mindfulness
- Vulnerability to mindlessness
- Tendency toward doubt, inquiry, and updating.
- Where mindfulness is most required
- Preoccupation with failure
- Reluctance to simplify
- Sensitivity to operations
- Commitment to resilience
- Deference to expertise in your firm

* (after Weick and Sutcliffe)

Table 10: Key strategies to build safer systems*

Enhance organisational mindfulness
- Preoccupation with failure; learn from mistakes, but look beyond the obvious for patterns and interconnections
- Enhance communication at and among all levels of the organisation

Promote organisational learning
- Avoid reliance upon the same success techniques that have worked in the past, but rather continually develop new methods
- Break down communication barriers

Simplify where possible and have sufficient, but not excessive redundancies

Enhance sensitivity to operations
- Develop and utilise mechanisms to detect the early warning signs of a crisis

Commit to resilience
- Integrate crisis management with other programmes; do not make it a separate programme
- Develop a culture of safety.

---

*based on Weick and Sutcliffe, Mitroff, West, Evan and Manion, Berniker and Wolf

12 | Personalised therapeutics impact on treatment efficiency

Stephen Guy

The application of *agility* concepts is not just for health care processes. The advancement of medicine technology is another means by which responsive and personalised care can be experienced by patients.

In 2001, **Celera Genomics** (Rockville, MD) published the 'human genome sequence', comprising 30,000 genes, based on samples from five individuals. Understanding the genetic alphabet does not provide enough information to make a drug. Now the emphasis is on studying gene function, gene expression, and genetic variations in healthy and diseased individuals.

The results of this research combined with the rapid rise of proteomics as a drug discovery technology is enabling biotech and pharmaceutical companies to consider 'personalised' drug development and therapy. According to industry forecasts, as drug developers wait 15 years for genomics-based therapeutics to come along, diagnostics culled from genomic data will have taken centre stage in just five.

Two kinds of molecular diagnostics will emerge from genomic research:

1. The first group will comprise tests for inherited disease, predisposition, and prenatal screening.
2. The second group will consist of new molecular tests for definitive diagnosis.

The first group will definitely need the physician to provide genetic counselling and interpretation for the individual. With the second group, the results will be binary, either you have a certain gene... or you do not.

As awareness grows that in the future primary-care health professionals will practise genomic medicine, how this will be

[i] Imai, M. *Gemba Kaizen.* McGraw-Hill, 1997

[ii] Tozawa B, *The idea generator: Quick and Easy Kaizen.* PCS Press, 2001.

[iii] Akao, Y, *Hoshin Kanri: Policy Deployment for successful TQM.* Productivity Press, 1991.

[iv] Babich P, *Hoshin Handbook.* Total Quality Engineering Inc, 1996.

[v] Crosby PB, *Quality is free*, Mentor Books, 1992.

achieved, and its impact on the efficiency of the treatment process needs to be considered.

To ensure a positive impact of these new technologies it is necessary to understand the characteristics of a lean, agile and efficient system, as summarised in Table 11:

Table 11 Characteristics of lean, agile systems

- High throughput
- Low cost
- Flexible
- High quality

These descriptions betray their production engineering origins and are familiar to managers and engineers working throughout the world in the manufacturing industry. The concept of lean, agile systems has been adopted by industry as a tool to compete globally, where speed to market and ability to continually adapt to change are essential for success, if not survival. Techniques such as Kaizen[i,ii] and Hoshin[iii,iv] have enhanced organisational and process efficiency, and quality initiatives such as Six-Sigma[v] towards improvements in product delivery and service.

The following sections consider how these characteristics map onto the proposed developments in molecular diagnostics and genomics-based therapeutics.

Molecular diagnostics

In the case of the first group of molecular diagnostics (tests for inherited disease, predisposition and prenatal screening), the physician will need to invest significant time in explaining the tests and counselling the patient on the results. The pairing of screening tests with a corresponding treatment regime or counselling is necessary to avoid patients experiencing a sense of despair.

The overall efficiency of the treatment process will increase provided that sufficient numbers of patients follow the recommendations of the physician, reducing further consultations and medication. Critical to the success in directing patients to follow a certain treatment regime, or make changes to lifestyle, is the counselling skill of the physician and the ability to communicate risks. It is likely that an increase in screening will encourage patients to consider their own risk factors rather than those of the associated group, where there is an inherent degree of uncertainty and applicability. The selection of drug therapies based on information gained from molecular diagnostics on efficacy and predisposition to side effects will also emphasis the concept of personalised risk. Health care providers will also need to ensure that training of physicians is maintained at a sufficient level to counsel patients adequately and to provide the tools to communicate risk effectively.

Other initiatives that could be taken include:

* Use genomic screening statistical data to give the patient an accurate assessment of risks, particularly, if recommended changes to lifestyle, or adherence to the treatment regime are not followed
* For health care providers to make treatments selectively available based on patients taking personal responsibility for changes to lifestyle, or adherence to treatment regimes.
* Life assurance and pension providers structuring premiums on the basis of the patients agreeing to adopt the recommended therapeutic regime.

Additionally, the first group of molecular diagnostics could also improve the efficiency of the treatment process, by identifying trends in disease within the population and geographically. Health care providers will then be in a better position to target resources where they are most needed.

The second group of molecular diagnostics (providing a definite diagnosis) potentially offers improvements to treatment efficiency, as physicians will be able to apply the most effective treatment earlier. It will provide physicians with precise information that helps them select the most appropriate treatment from those currently available, and also may broaden the application of specific drugs. This type of diagnostic tool also offers considerable benefits in the drug discovery process as a method of testing targeted drugs. The difficulties with this form of molecular diagnostics are the complex nature of disease and the multiplicity of factors that need to be considered in making a diagnosis. As an example of the complexity, when developing molecular diagnostics for cancer it is necessary to look at the cancer genome as a separate entity, and then look at the patient or host themselves. A question also remains for the physician to decide on an individual basis whether or not early diagnosis of disease is beneficial for the patient.

Table 12: Treatment process improvements offered by developments in molecular diagnostics

Characteristics of lean, agile systems	Compatibility with developments in molecular screening.	Comments
Higher throughput	Yes	Given that patients use the information provided to make good health care choices.
Lower cost	Yes	Positive diagnosis offers efficient use of medication. Screening statistics enable health care providers to target patient needs more effectively.
Increased flexibility	Yes	'Personalised screening' addresses the needs of the individual rather than the collective.
Improved quality	Yes	Genomic-based screening accurate and repeatable.

Quality, if defined as 'Conformance to Requirements', will be enhanced due to accuracy and repeatability of molecular diagnostic screening based on genomics.

The potential offered by developments in molecular diagnostics to deliver improvements to the treatment process is summarised in Table 12.

Genomics-based therapeutics

The patient's reluctance to follow a recommended drug treatment regime is often a result, or fear of side effects. Genomics-based therapeutics offers the potential for 'personalised' drugs where the medication is extremely effective, and will present minimal side effects. Treatment throughput will be increased by the effectiveness of the therapy and its acceptance by patients, and costs of medication will be reduced through the reduction in side effects.

The *agility* of the treatment process will also increase as therapies become tailored to the needs of the individual rather than the collective. Quality will be enhanced as '*Personalised*' drugs conform closer to the ideal requirements for a therapeutic drug, being effective and exhibiting little if any side effects. And here we see agility in action, where the patient is treated as an individual rather than as part of a mass customised process.

The potential offered by developments in genomics-based therapeutics to deliver lean, agile improvements in the treatment process, is summarised in Table 13.

Table 13: Treatment process improvements offered by developments in genomics-based therapeutics

Characteristics of lean, agile systems	Compatibility with developments in genomics-based therapeutics	Comments
Higher throughput	Yes	Targeted drugs optimise drug performance and effectiveness. Patient acceptance of treatment is enhanced by minimising side effects.
Lower cost	Yes	Effectiveness of drug and reduced side effects lowers costs.
Increased flexibility	Yes	'Personalised drugs' address the needs of the individual rather than the collective.
Increased quality	Yes	Conform closer to the ideal requirements for a therapeutic drug.

Discussion

Genomics offers the opportunity for a more powerful and economical form of preventative medicine allowing each of us to establish an effective programme of diet, life style, and medical surveillance to diminish our risk of future illness. It promises to allow a better determination of which drugs to give to which individual, increasing efficacy and reducing side effects.

As an example of how developments in this field are progressing, in September 2001, the Food and Drug Administration (FDA) approved the TRUEGENE HIV-1 Genotyping Kit and OpenGene DNA Sequencing System. This product is for use in detecting HIV genomic mutations that confer resistance to specific types of anti-retroviral drugs, as an aid in monitoring and treating HIV infection.

Key to the development and deployment of genomics technologies are the opportunities available for commercial exploitation and the investment required. Early pointers indicate that this technology will lead to a re-distribution in costs, benefiting the front-end health care and treatment process. Lending support to this view, it has recently been reported that a large not-for-profit health care network in the US has embarked on a collaborative programme on the large-scale application of clinical genetic testing to patient care. Initially focussing on the prediction of cardiovascular disease, it is planned that individualised patient care plans will be based on the screening results. An aim of the work is for it to become a model for implementation at large integrated health care systems.

Biotechnology and pharmaceutical companies are seeing that having access to too much genomics data can be as confounding as having too little. Significant investment will therefore be necessary in integrating and sharing information among the myriad sources of bioinformatic data and developing bioinformatic tools.

Additionally, to realise the concept of 'Personalised' drugs, even if these are for groups of patients rather than individuals, will require significant investment in the development of automated systems for drug discovery and delivery.

Enabling technologies are being discovered in the fields of DNA extraction and replication and storage. There are a variety of technologies that are being applied to the development of molecular-based tests. These include hybridisation, real-time polymerase chain reaction, and sequencing-based technologies. Fermentation and cell culturing technology is of interest because it makes it possible to mass-produce a number of natural products of commercial importance at relatively low cost.

Equally important will be the availability of automated technologies that can identify genetic alterations and then screen for their presence in large populations.

It is interesting to note that to realise the full potential of 'Personalised' therapeutics will require automated processes that exhibit the same characteristics as lean and agile systems.

13 | Policy implications

Barry Tennison, Nigel Edwards

Introduction

This book has highlighted the advantages of agility in health care, and some of the ways in which health care organisations and systems can become more agile – that is, flexible and adaptable. But how can policy at national and local level be designed to promote agility and support an environment in which it can prosper? This chapter addresses this question, mainly for the NHS in the UK. It also has implications for the policies pursued within health care organisations, for example concerning the ways their staff are treated; and how that performance is managed.

Principles derived from what we know about agility

Previous chapters have emphasised a number of features of agile systems and organisations. Some of the factors which encourage or discourage agility, as derived from the rest of the book, are given in Box 10.

Agile systems are complex adaptive systems. Small changes can have a large impact on the whole of the system, without there being the possibility of predicting what might happen. Alternatively, the converse is often seen, where large-scale changes have little impact. Change can arise spontaneously out of a disorganised or apparently destructive or tense situation. This can result in new and innovative ways of working. In particular, individuals or groups in agile systems can resist change, or bring about large-scale change, depending on the nature of the system, and most crucially on:

- its degree of interconnectedness
- the nature of the control mechanisms
- its capacity to learn and adapt.

Box 10: Agility – encouragers and discouragers

The following are elements or factors which tend to enhance agility:

- clarity of purpose, focus and commitment
- ability to actively manage knowledge
- active collaborative learning
- feedback from the environment
- the existence of 'slack', capacity to experiment and take on new approaches
- team working and good team relationships
- good working across boundaries
- attention to the 'shadow system' of informal relationships, gossip and rumour
- developing personal and organisational capability
- enabled co-evolution.

The following are elements or factors which tend to inhibit or impair agility:

- oversimplifying
- rigid organisational design
- rigid process design
- performance measurement used with deterrent effects
- degrees of rigid control.

To encourage organisations and systems to be increasingly agile, policy should help the positive factors to flourish, and inhibit or control the negative factors (see Box 11).

The policy context

There are a number of significant drivers, in the UK and world-wide, that require health care organisations to be much more agile. These include:

- increasing consumerism, a reduced willingness to simply defer to professional opinion, supported by improved access to medical information by consumers
- pressures for cost containment from payers in most systems
- a much greater focus on quality and responsiveness
- fast moving clinical innovation and mushrooming amounts of new information from research.

Box 11: How policy can inhibit agility

A health organisation in the UK set up reasonably robust mechanisms to discuss priorities openly with stakeholders in its local population. This led to an explicit policy about low priority treatments, which included in vitro fertilisation (IVF) as being not normally supported.

Some potential patients, in sensible discussion and negotiation with the organisation, offered to pay part of the cost of the treatment if the organisation would pay the rest. The organisation would like to have agreed to this, as part of its attempts to meet population expectations in a flexible way (an aspect of agility).

However, national policy in the UK prohibits any co-payments by NHS patients beyond those (like prescription charges) that are a statutory part of the system. The health organisation was therefore not able to agree to the compromise. It had to fund the whole treatment, or not at all.

National policy on co-payments for NHS patients reflects political views on equity and the principle that the NHS is 'free at the point of delivery' (with very restricted exceptions). National policy inhibited agility in this case.

A significant problem is that government and others in charge of complex hierarchical systems tend to approach policy making and the management of performance in ways that may actually discourage the development of agility. These are covered in the next few sections, and include ideology; models of change; policy making processes; risk aversion; a simplistic view of efficiency; and the view taken of the overall system.

Ideology

It is important to distinguish ideology from the norms and values of an organisation or its vision or purpose. Ideology is the set of beliefs underpinning a theory, usually political, whereas the norms, values, objectives and mission of organisations tend to be pragmatic rather than based on a particular theoretical or ideological standpoint.

In a recent conference paper Professor Calum Paton argued that ideology is still significant in underpinning policy making despite what he describes as the increasingly negotiable nature of ideology at the margin and the move from 'there is no alternative' to 'what matters is what works'. Ideology or belief systems about the best approach are very powerful and whilst policy makers may believe that they are simply acting on evidence this may be

137

significantly influenced by being seen through the lens of a particular ideology. It would be a mistake to believe that these are not
also at work in apparently more pragmatic environments such as
manufacturing but they are much more overt, pervasive and powerful in politically influenced areas such as health care. Ideology is
a significant handicap to the adoption of agile practices because it
encompasses ideas about both what should be done and how it
should be accomplished. In doing so ideology has the power to
shut down the thinking, learning and adaptive processes needed
for successful agility. It also tends to move the focus from the customer or end user to the ideology itself or at least to its main pro-
ponents – politicians, political advisors and some academics.

The ideological basis of much policy making leads to an
assumption that there is a shared or common domain of dis-
course; that doctors, nurses, other front line staff, managers and
(in the UK) the Department of Health share a similar set of objectives, values, and ways of thinking. This is not necessarily true and
in fact the ideology of hierarchy itself is somewhat questionable in
health care as the top of the organisation is often disconnected
from the front line.

Models of change

Policy makers and politicians tend to have a simplistic and linear
model of change management. This may be because in politics the
predominant model is one in which heroic style leaders issue com-
mands which are picked up and implemented by others. Without
the glue of ideology the transfer of this model to real life often
requires central control and a system which is reliant on very
detailed targets supported by inspection, standards and carrots
and sticks. The approach is somewhat unitary and managerialist
in that the implications of pluralism are downplayed and opposi-
tion is characterised as unreasonable.

The first problem with this is that prescriptive centrally
designed policies have insufficient regard to variations in starting
points or other local contexts and contingencies that have potentially enormous implications for the success of the policy. At its
most absurd this has resulted in national targets being allocated on
a simple share basis between areas; for example in the decisions
about the purchase of new CT scanners.

A second problem is that the insight that targets can produce
change is erroneously generalised to the conclusion that more targets will produce more change and that interim targets will ensure

forward movement. Underpinning this is a view that without this discipline there will be no way of ensuring progress. This partly seems to come from the need to equip ministers with the means to demonstrate progress and partly from a tendency to suspect that left to their own devices the front line would do little to implement change.

In addition to targets, there has been much reliance on incentives and structural changes as a method of dealing with the failure to meet objectives which results from the disconnected hierarchy found in most health care organisations. Reliance on these methods fails to give appropriate weight to the problems of dysfunctional relationships and information exchange that often underlie many of these issues.

There are particular problems associated with a hierarchical conception of the organisation or system in which ideas can be 'driven down' by traditional implementation methods. In fact in many cases the hierarchy is at best disconnected and at worst conceptualised and experienced very differently by front line staff. This is exacerbated by the model of clinical management often having been seen as being advocate, protector and securer of resources rather than strong participant in a corporate and collective endeavour.

Policy making processes

A particular issue for the development of agility is a model of policy making which prefers policy to be designed rather than grown through experiment and testing. Indeed the term pilot in the NHS very often is a euphemism for phase 1 of a roll out programme. There is limited use of policy evaluation and indeed there is little formal evaluation of even quite significant policy changes. This has its roots in a reductionist approach that tends to aim to produce well designed policies for individual parts of the system. Unfortunately the implications of complexity, feedback loops and the non-additive nature of policy means that this will not necessarily produce a satisfactory overall set of policies.

A second problem for the development of agility lies in the risk aversion and the short termism produced by electoral timescales and the effect of politics that tends to deny or obscure failure rather than using it as an opportunity to learn. Learning from diversity is also inhibited by a tendency to see it as an indictment of the system – 'unacceptable variation' – rather than a necessary part of innovation and agility.

A third problem in the UK is that policy makers have adopted a view of efficiency that has a bias against redundancy, flexible capacity and which has mistaken cheapness for efficiency. For example, until recently the prevailing orthodoxy was that target average occupancy for NHS hospitals should be close to 90% for acute wards, whereas it is likely that lower levels of occupancy are necessary for high quality and flexibility of care.

Policy makers' view of the system

In addition to the misunderstanding about the disconnected nature of hierarchies in health care, there is an assumption (in the teeth of the evidence) that power is something that is held centrally and devolved or granted to others, rather than being much more likely to be vested in front line staff who have a long tradition of autonomy.

This set of belief tends to support an approach to policy making in which the centre or top of the system is seen as having a superior view of what is required and a special role in providing instructions to other parts to ensure co-ordination. This has particular implications for setting targets and the collection of information. We noted the tendency to set a plethora of targets. In addition there is the problem that it is assumed that targets that seem reasonable when set nationally will be appropriate when translated to local organisations. The collection of information by the centre to feed this process can become very onerous. Inspectors and civil servants ask 'how can you manage your organisation unless you know ...'. Unfortunately this ignores the reality that the answer usually is 'quite easily'. The management of key staff in any organisation that wants to come even close to agility can rely on tight numerical targets only for a relatively small number of indicators. Mostly they will rely on individual accountability across a range of areas which are continually monitored, adjusted and reinforced by a series of conversations within the framework of an overall direction rather than a large number of detailed targets. The current approach to policy and performance management may be making the mistake of treating individuals as if they were organisations.

The current approach to information collection for performance management also produces incentives to manipulate the answers that are given and the process may severely detract from the focus required to deliver the goals that are really important. All of these features of the system represent a significant obstacle to the development of new ways of working or the type of agility that we would wish to see develop.

Policy implications

A policy framework which would foster agility needs to be able to create the pressure to respond to the customer in an environment in which typically there is a third party payer and the end user often has their demand mediated through an agent who may be an employee or subcontractor. This is different from the usual situation in manufacturing or most service industries. In those systems where the government is the payer and the manager of the provider side, there is an additional set of complications which can significantly undermine agility other than the requirement to meet government targets (or show that they appear to have been met). This has led to a number of recent suggestions that the NHS should be removed from direct political control. If agility is about being able to rapidly respond to the needs of customers this proposal does not address the fundamental confusion about who the customer actually is. Nevertheless, there are some things that would promote the development of a policy framework to support the development of more agile health care organisations.

Policy needs to build an environment that makes space for creativity, and removes or minimises the disincentives to experiment and rules that dampen imagination, ingenuity and inventiveness. This will allow those who run organisations, and in particular their middle managers, to find ways to harness the available resourcefulness, particularly of people who work directly with patients. This entails some significant risks and will require a number of important changes in the overall approach to policy and performance management which are considered below.

A second important measure would be to encourage the cross-fertilisation of ideas, both within the organisation and outside (for example, encouraging staff to become members of peer review teams that review other organisations) to promote learning and innovation. An important aspect of this would be the development of new ways to involve patients and prospective patients in a dialogue about the design and operation of the services they use.

Whilst procedures and protocols have their place in ensuring that care for complex but relatively predictable conditions is made more systematic, they have to be used in a way that does not compromise the development of creativity and consumer responsiveness. Once a decision has been made to depart from the well trodden path of protocols and procedures, one of the most difficult changes is to allow front line staff and local leaders to take risks and to manage the effects when they go wrong. The consequences of innovation are often unpredictable, and a relatively long time may be needed to evaluate its effects. Not only are policy makers (and especially politicians) risk averse, they also are prone to short-termism and a tendency to attribute blame to individuals. All of these features are inimical to the development of agility. The role particularly for local managers is to find ways to create protected space to allow for risk taking and innovation and to have the ability to wait for results. This may mean taking steps to encourage self-organisation by setting overall direction, granting permissions, creating space and being very clear on the small number of absolutely non-negotiable must-dos.

The policy framework will need to support this with a number of measures that:

- encourage thinking 'outside the box', rather than continuing past practice or slavish imitation of others
- create incentives and consequences which encourage innovation, creativity and appropriate risk taking
- avoid rigidity in the processes for performance management
- build capacity in organisations and skills in those that lead them to support this.

The implications of this are that many planning processes will need to be rethought. In particular the idea that rational planning will necessarily bring about the intended results, rather than the unintended consequences found in complex adaptive systems, will need to be continually questioned.

Conclusion

Survival and sustainability of health care systems and organisations depend on their capacity to evolve, and to co-evolve with other elements of the social world. Agility may well be needed to ensure this.

Policies can encourage or discourage the development and improvement of agile systems but there are some unique aspects of the health care policy environment that have the potential to undermine this. Given the complex adaptive nature of health care systems and organisations, those setting policies should have an understanding of:

- the constraints on the effectiveness of policies
- which sorts of policies are likely to encourage or discourage agility.

In the increasingly complex world, it is likely that inappropriate policies, stifling agility, will lead to failure or atrophy of health care systems and organisations.

References

Akao Y, *Hoshin Kanri: Policy Deployment for successful TQM.* Productivity Press, 1991.

Armstrong M, Baron A, *Performance Management: The New Realities*, Institute of Personnel and Development, London, 1998.

Ashkenas R, Ulrich D, Jick T, Kerr S, *The Boundaryless Organisation:Breaking the Chains of Organisational Structure*, San Francisco, Jossey Bass, 1995.

Babich P, *Hoshin Handbook.* Total Quality Engineering Inc, 1996.

Berniker E, Wolf F, *Managing Complex Technical Systems Working on a Bridge of Uncertainty* http://www.plu.edu/~bernike/ManComSys/ Managing%20ComplexSystemsIAMOT.doc accessed July 8, 2002.

Berwick D, 'Run to space' Address to the National Forum for Health care Improvement, 1995 (6 Dec).

Binns P, The Change Agile Organisation. www.ie.edu/efmd/ documents/The_Agile_Organisation.ppt accessed April 17, 2002.

Bristol Inquiry. Available online at http://www.bristol-inquiry.org.uk/.

Cheng TCE, Podolsky S, *Just-in-Time Manufacturing – an Introduction*, Chapman & Hall, London, 1993.

Crosby PB, *Quality is free*, Mentor Books, 1992.

Department of Health, *The NHS Plan: a Plan for Investment : a Plan for Reform*, HMSO, 2000 (July).

Department of Health, *Shifting the Balance of Power within the NHS – Securing Delivery*, London, HMSO, 2001 (July).

Department of Health, *The NHS Plan: A plan for investment: A plan for reform*, London HMSO, 2001 (July).

Dove R, Design Principles for Highly Adaptable Business Systems, With Tangible Manufacturing Examples, www.parshift.com, 1999.

Dove R, 'Knowledge management, response ability, and the agile enterprise', *Journal of Knowledge Management*, 3(1), 1999, pp. 18–35.

Ibid., p. 18.

Dove R. *Design Principles for Highly Adaptable Business Systems, With Tangible Manufacturing Examples.* www.parshift.com/docs/ RrsPrinciplesMIH.htm accessed July 8, 2002.

Drucker PF, *Management: Tasks, Responsibilities, Practices*, Heinemann, London, 1974.

Encarta World English Dictionary, Microsoft Corporation, 1999.

Ibid.

Evan WM, Manion M, *Minding the Machines: Preventing Technological Disasters*. Prentice Hall PTR, Upper Saddle River, New Jersey, 2002.

Forrester JW, *Industrial Dynamics*, MIT Press: Cambridge, 1961.

Fraser SW, Burch K, Knightley M, Osborne M, Wilson A, 'Using collaborative improvement in a single organisation: improving anticoagulant care', *International Journal for Health Care Quality Assurance*, 15(4, 5), 2002.

Fraser SW, Greenhalgh T, Complexity science: coping with complexity: educating for capability. *BMJ* 323:799–803, 2001.

Fraser SW, *The Patient's Journey; 35 Tools for Mapping, Analysing and Improving Health care Processes*, Kingsham Press, Chichester, UK, 2002.

Freeman AC, Sweeney K, Why general practitioners do not implement evidence: qualitative study, *BMJ*; 323: 1100, 2001.

Freeman T, Using performance indicators to improve health care quality in the public sector: a review of the literature. *Health Services Management Research* 15: 126–137, 2002.

Goldman SL, Graham CB, *Agility in Health Care: Strategies for Mastering Turbulent Markets*, San Francisco, Jossey Bass, 1999.

Goldman SL, Agile competitors and virtual organizations: strategies for enriching the customer, Van Nostrand Reinhold, 1994 (cited in Robertson, M and Jones, C, Application of lean production and agile manufacturing concepts in a telecommunications environment, *International Journal of Agile Management Systems*, 1(1), 1999).

Goldman SL, Graham C (eds) *Agility in Health Care: Strategies for Mastering Turbulent Markets*. Jossey-Bass, 1999.

Ibid.

Goldratt E, 'Focusing on constraints, not costs'. In *Rethinking the Future*, edited by Gibson R, Nicholas Brierly Publishing, London, 1998.

Goldratt EM, Cox J, *The Goal*, Gower, Aldershot, 1984.

Goldratt EM, *What is this Thing Called Theory of Constraints and How Should it be Implemented?* Croton-on-Hudson, N.Y.: North River Press, 1990.

goodpractice.net, *Performance management – Effective Management Practice – Good Practice: AA Insurance*, www.goodpractice.net, 24th March 2002.

goodpractice.net, *Performance management – Effective management practice – Good Practice: Volkswagen*, www.goodpractice.net, 24th March 2002.

goodpractice.net, *The Importance of Performance Management – an Overview*, www.goodpractice.net, 24th March 2002.

Hanson P, Voss CA, Blackmon K, Oak, B, *Made in Europe, A Four Nations Best Practice Study*, IBM UK Ltd/London Business School, Warwick/London, 1994.

Imai, M. *Gemba Kaizen*. McGraw-Hill, 1997.

Institute for Health care Improvement, Boston, Mass, 1995 www.ihi.org.

Investors in People, *Investors in People: The context*,
www.iipuk.co.uk/investorsinpople/thestandard/, 18th October 2002.

Kanter RM, *When Giants Learn to Dance*, London, International
Thomson Business Press, 1998.

Kaplan R, Norton D, 'Balanced Scorecard: measures that drive
performance', *Harvard Business Review*, January–February 1992.

Kiesler S, Spoull L, 'Reducing social context clues: electronic mail in
organisational communication' in: *Connections New Ways of Working
in the Networked Organisation*, Cambridge, MIT Press, 1986.

Kostner J, *Virtual Leadership*, London, Warner Business Books, 1996.

Lipnack J, Stamps J, *Virtual Teams*, New York, John Wiley, 2000.

Locock L, *Maps and Journeys; Redesign in the NHS*, HSMC
Birmingham, 2001.

Maskell, B 'The Journey to Agile Manufacturing', www.maskell.com.

McNutt R, Abrams R, Aron DC for the Patient Safety Committee.
Patient safety efforts should focus on medical errors. *JAMA*
287:1997–2001, 2002.

Metes G, Gundry J, Bradish P, *Agile Networking*, Prentice Hall PTR,
1998.

Modernisation Agency, *Ideal Design of Emergency Access (IDEA)
Programme: National Report*, Modernisation Agency, 2002
(January).

Monden Y, *Toyota Production System – Practical Approach to Production
Management*, Industrial Engineering and Management Press,
Norcorss, Georgia, 1983.

Morden T, Principles of Management, London, McGraw-Hill, 1996.

Mullan F, A Founder of Quality Assessment Encounters a troubled
system firsthand. Shortly before his death, Avedis Donabedian
talked with about health care and the management of his own
cancer care. *Health Affairs*, 20(1); 137–142, 2001.

Murray M, 'Patient Care: Access', *BMJ*, 320:1594–1596, 2000.

National Audit Office, *Inappropriate adjustments to NHS waiting lists*.
London: The Stationery Office, 2001.

Neely A, *Measuring Business Performance – Why, What and How*, Profile
Books Ltd., London, 1998, p. 1.

Ibid., p. 3.

Pedler M, Issues in health development: networked organisations – an
overview, NHS Development Agency: www.had-online.org.uk, 2001.

Perrow C, *Normal Accidents*. New York, Basic Books, 1999.

Pidgeon N, The Limits to Safety? Culture, Politics, Learning and Man-
Made Disasters. *Journal of Contingencies and Crises Management*
55(1), March 1997.

Plsek PE, Greenhalgh P, The challenge of complexity in health care, *BMJ*, 323:625–8, 2001.

Reason J, *Managing the Risks of Organizational Accidents*. Aldershot, UK, Ashgate Publishing Ltd., 1997.

Richmond B, 'Systems Thinking: Critical Thinking Skills for the 1990s and beyond'. *Systems Dynamics Review* 9(2), 113–133, 1993.

Robinson D, Hewitt T, Harris J (eds), *Managing Development; Understanding Inter-organizational Relationships*, Sage: London, 2000.

Sackett D, Haynes B, Tugwell P, Guyatt G, Clinical Epidemiology: A Basic Science for Clinical Medicine. Hagerstown, MD USA. Lippincott Williams & Wilkins Publishers, 1991.

Schonberger RJ, *World Class Manufacturing – the Lessons of Simplicity Applied*, The Free Press, New York, 1986.

Sharifi H, Zhang Z, Agile Manufacturing in Practice Application of a Methodology, *International Journal of Operations and Production Management*, 21(5/6), pp 772–794, 2001.

Slack N, Chambers S, Harland C, Harrison A, Johnston R, *Operations Management*, Pitman Publishing, London, 1995, pp. 628–629.

Smith P, The unintended consequences of publishing performance data in the public sector. *International Journal of Public Administration* 18(2): 277–310, 1995.

Stacey R, *Strategic Management and Organisational Dynamics; the challenge of complexity*, 3rd Edition London: Financial Times, 1999.

Stahr H, Bulman B, Stead M, *The Excellence Model in Healthcare*, Chichester, Kingsham Press, 2000.

Stephenson J, 'Capability and quality in higher education' in Stephenson J, York M, eds. *Capability and Quality in Higher Education*, Kogan-Page, London, 1995.

Taylor FW, 'Shop Management' in *Scientific Management*, Harper & Row: USA, 1964 (original article written in 1911).

The future of UK's family doctors: new contract: www.bma.org.uk/ap.nsf/Content/_Hub+GPC+contract.

Tozawa B, *The idea generator: Quick and Easy Kaizen*. PCS Press, 2001.

Vaughan D, *The Challenger Launch Decision*. Chicago, University of Chicago Press, 1996.

Weick K, Sutcliffe K, Quinn R, *Managing the Unexpected: Assuring High Performance in an Age of Complexity*. San Francisco. Jossey-Bass, 2001.

West E, Organisational sources of safety and danger: sociological contributions to the study of adverse events. *Quality in Health Care* 9:120–126, 2000.

Wheatley M, *Leadership and the New Science*. Berrett-Koehler Publishers Inc, 2001.

Womack JP, Jones DT, *Lean Thinking*, Touchstone Books, London, 1996.

Womack JP, Jones DT, *Lean Thinking: Banish Waste and Create Wealth in your Corporation*, Touchstone Books, London, 1998.

Zimmerman, B Lindberg, C, Plsek P, *Edgeware; Insights from Complexity Science for Health care Leaders*, Texas: VHA Inc, 1998.

Index